NATURALLY HEALTHY HAIR

Herbal Treatments and Daily Care for Fabulous Hair

MARY BETH JANSSEN

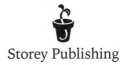

Storey Publishing

The mission of Storey Publishing is to serve our
customers by publishing practical information that encourages
personal independence in harmony with the environment.

Edited by Deborah Balmuth and Nancy Ringer
Text design by Carol Jessop, Black Trout Design
Text production by Susan B. Bernier and Jennifer Jepson Smith
Cover art & design by Carol Jessop
Line drawings by Alison Kolesar
Spot illustrations by Laura Tedeschi
Indexed by Peggy Holloway

Printed in the United States by Edwards Brothers, Inc.
10 9 8 7 6 5 4 3

Library of Congress Cataloging-in-Publication Data

Janssen, Mary Beth.
    Naturally healthy hair : herbal treatments and daily care for fabulous hair / Mary Beth Janssen.
        p.   cm.
    Includes bibliographical references and index.
    ISBN 1-58017-129-X (pbk. : alk. paper)
    1. Hair—Care and hygiene.   2. Medicine, Ayurvedic.   3. Hair preparations.   I. Title.
    RL91.J36   1999
    646.7'24—dc21   99-33058
                                                                        CIP

DEDICATION

To God, for showing me the way of love. To the light and love of my life, Jim. You are always there supporting me in all my endeavors, but most importantly you make me laugh, and lightheartedness is what it is all about. Thanks for your unconditional love. To my wonderful family, and especially my mother and father, Nelly and Hubert. You are the most incredible inspiration! And you have been my best teachers. I have truly been blessed with you as my loving parents.

ACKNOWLEDGMENTS

I wish to acknowledge Storey Publishing for their commitment to natural health and beauty — and would like to especially thank Nancy Ringer and Deborah Balmuth for their inspired editorial guidance.

Thank you to all my creative colleagues, teachers, and friends who have been such an important part of my evolution: my mentors, Leo Passage from Pivot Point International and Vi Nelson from Vi Nelson and Associates — you truly are an Executive Goddess; Deepak Chopra, M.D., David Simon, M.D., Nan Johnson, Roger Gabriel, Jenny Hatheway, and the entire Chopra organization; Dr. Christiane Northrup, Bea Sochor, Leslie Pace, Susan MacLeary, Judy Rambert, Mary Atherton, Gordon Miller, Grace and Buddy Francis, Teresa Pupillo, Luis Romero, Linda Burmeister, Carlos Valenzuela, Xenon, Dwight Miller, David Raccuglia, Lawrence Hegarty, Brian Fallon, Elsa Harolds, Glyn Jones, Patrick Kalle, Jan Laan, James Koktavy, Lynn Maestro, Bianca Simball, Althea Northage-Orr, Patricia Howell, Professor Steven Zdatny, Melanie Sachs, Rachel Geller, Bob Seidl, Ben Polk, and Pamela Lappies; Marlene Hansen from the International Association of Trichologists; and Denise Santamarina from The Natural Nouveaux Salon.

Thank you to my wonderful friends from *Modern Salon, American Salon,* and *Salon News,* Advanstar IBS, the Chicago Cosmetologists Association, the National Cosmetologists Association, the Salon Association, the Fashion Group International, Delmar Publishing, and the Himalayan Institute, and to all of my clients, past, present, and future, who are seeking to live a more holistic lifestyle and put their trust in me. And last but not least, thanks to all my students. I truly believe that "by learning you will teach; by teaching you will learn." You have all been awe-inspiring.

CONTENTS

CHAPTER 1
Understanding Hair Culture
▼▼▼

$\mathcal{S}$ince time immemorial, human beings have been cognizant and appreciative of the meaning attached to the grooming and appearance of their hair. It can affect us deeply as a source of pure delight and intrigue or as an absolute repulsion. Around the world, and specifically in the United States where we spend billions of dollars every year trying to control our hair, we cut, comb, brush, condition, color, curl, slick, spray, and grow to convey a style that has a language all its own. Think, for example, of the expectations a beauty pageant contestant has for her hair versus those of of a female corporate executive. Thanks to the history of hair culture, we've been taught to assign vastly different meanings to different hairstyles.

Hair is a visual record of the incredible diversity of people around the planet, and it represents a richness of worldwide cultures that is slowly but surely shrinking as globalization encourages worldwide conformity to the norms of Western cultures or "developed" countries. Whether the elaborately magnificent hairstyles of the Fulani women of northern Guinea (which signify different stages of their lives), the intricate and time-consuming braids of the Senegalese women, or the Rastafarians' dreadlocks (which signify their devotion to their God), the importance of hairstyles in the expression of a culture is undeniable. A sumo wrestler's topknot is so integral to the spiritual nature of his sporting life that it is ceremoniously cut off upon retirement. In Cambodia, bride and groom have ceremonial haircuts during the wedding to ward off evil influences that may unduly affect the newlyweds. From Dominican friars to Buddhist monks, many spiritual supplicants remove their hair to symbolize renunciation of all earthly attachments.

Depending on where your travels take you, your hair may not only be the subject of strong prejudices, it could also be a crime — long hair on men is banned in Malaysia, while a clean-cut look in the northern Indian state of Punjab could

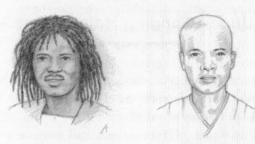

Rastafarian dreadlocks   A monk's shaved head

get you killed. Women unveiling their long hair in strict Islamic countries face a jail sentence, while women of a certain Mexican tribe are ostracized for cutting their hair short. Corn-row braids can get you expelled from some U.S. schools, and disobeying strict corporate dress codes, whether by growing your hair long, shaving your scalp, or perhaps wearing highly unnatural hair colors, can get you fired.

The nature of hair has continuously evolved through civilizations and cultures, but regardless of time or place, one thing holds true: Our perception creates our reality. Our feelings of self-worth and self-esteem thus build the attitude we hold toward our own hair, and the attractiveness quotient we attach to the way we style it.

THE HISTORY OF HAIRSTYLING

Cultural ideals of hair have continued to change and evolve throughout history in tandem with the hopes, dreams, trials, and glories of the times. Even though a hairstyle may have been considered the most appealing at the time, it was not always the healthiest or the most natural expression of beauty. If in medieval times the rage was to wear incredibly ornate wigs over a clean-shaven scalp that went unwashed for lengthy periods of time, then so be it. It was the accepted norm at the time.

The earliest Egyptians for the most part let their hair grow long, wavy, and free, and paid very little attention to it, until at some point in time an inspired individual decided that hair was entirely too much of a bother. Thus began the ancient Egyptian fashion for both men and women to shave their heads and don wigs. This caught on to such a degree that an entire industry of barbers and wig makers was born to keep all Egyptian heads adorned with elaborate headdresses and hairpieces. Natural hair was despised, so much so that decrees were written to make the shaving of all natural hair a part of religion.

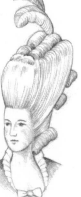

A typical Egyptian wig

Wigs also came to be tremendously popular in the ancient Roman Empire. That fashion was undermined for a brief time by the Caesar's legionnaires, who marched off into war with faces freshly shaved and hair clean cut and short. Eventually, when the Roman Empire split, the hair kingdom of men was divided as well, with the West adopting a clean-cut, shaven look and Eastern societies keeping their long hair and beards. Women of the ancient Roman Empire became bolder in showing the true nature of their natural hair, which had been either hidden away and disguised by all forms of hairpieces or kept covered in accord with the Church's admonitions not to arouse prurient sexual interest in men.

It is this dizzying back-and-forth nature of hair fashion through the centuries, and the generational rifts created by intense and complex arguments over the long and short of hair, that make the study of hair throughout history so fascinating.

Throughout the 18th century, America was a land of bewigged and hairpieced men and woman. Much of this fashion was brought over on the ships from Europe. And I must say that the styles of this period were less than natural and less than healthy. Women's extravagantly oversized and in many cases grotesque wigs were a craze among the general public. The hairdressers of the time were on call to create, freshen up, and in essence maintain what by today's standards would be considered monstrosities of nature. These wigs were wired and rigged and stuffed with all form of architectural paraphernalia to allow them to stand erect. The woman who wore them had to have supportive structures built in as well as special sleeping arrangements, because these "hairstyles"

Typical 18th-century elaborately styled wig

were intended to stay intact anywhere from two weeks to two months. It became a contest to see who could have designed and then wear the most awe-inspiring, and sometimes frightening, headdress! Ships were built, gardens were planted, solar systems revolved, all within the confines of the wig atop a woman's head — I kid you not.

A CENTURY OF STYLES

With the dawning of the 20th century, hairstyles started to take on, by today's standards, normalcy. Women wanted long hair, period. In fact, many forms of snake oil were sold to women anxious to grow the longest, most luxurious hair ever. "A woman's crowning glory is her hair" was the slogan used to sell a wide variety of hair growth elixirs and scalp cleaners. This was perhaps revolutionary, in that women began to pay attention to the God-given hair growing on their heads instead of all forms of fakery. Along with this attention came a keen interest in all forms of lotions, potions, and cosmetic means to keep the hair attractive. This is indeed the time when shampooing became more regular. The tide was beginning to turn toward more natural and healthy hairstyles.

The Gibson Girl

At about this same time, the artist Charles Dana Gibson penned an illustration of his dream girl, the Gibson Girl, who was destined to become the 20th century's first pinup. She created a sensation among men, and soon women around the world were looking to emulate this vision of femininity, loveliness, approachability, and liberation. Her pompadour was a loosely gathered-up style in which the hair was rolled and placed at the top of the head; soft tendrils were allowed to fall provocatively around the face and neck; think of Katharine Ross in *Butch Cassidy and the Sundance Kid.* The Gibson Girl was idealized as a woman who not only wore a sensuous and touchable hairstyle that exuded freedom, but would also hobnob with men on a variety of subjects of interest to them and, surprisingly enough, of interest to her.

At the same time Charles Gibson was creating a new mode in hair fashion for women, his illustrations included men adoringly surrounding their womanly vision, each of them with a debonair and quite clean-cut, clean-shaven look. (This style also extended to the clothing of the time.) These hairstyles for men would endure into the 1960s.

The Gibson Girl Pompadour

Traditionally, the pompadour is a loose, soft topknot, but many women today prefer a more tightly bound style, as shown here.

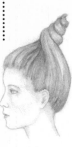

step 1

1. Gather all the lengths of hair up and out from the top of your head. Lightly twist the hair from its ends toward your scalp; don't twist too tightly.

2. Push the twisted hair toward your scalp area, making sure that the hair around the outer edges of the hairline is loose and full. Begin to form the twisted ends around themselves to form a soft topknot at the top of your head.

3. Pin the topknot in place to secure. Use a tail comb to adjust the volume around the outer edges and, if necessary, lightly backcomb and smooth shorter, looser hair into the style.

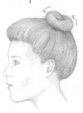

step 2

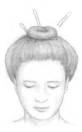

step 3

The Marcel Wave

With the invention of the marcel wave by French hairdresser Marcel Grateau, the American woman became bored with the pompadour. The marcel waving technique created sinuous, undulating waves in the hair worn down and around the head; think of Mia Farrow in *The Great Gatsby*. This technique is still used to create sultry waves, usually placed in mid- to long lengths of hair around the front hairline area to frame the face.

The traditional marcel wave (right) has evolved in popular culture to accommodate a short hairstyle as well (left).

The Permanent Wave

London hairdresser Charles Nessler invented the permanent wave in the early 20th century. This would further revolutionize hairstyles for women, allowing them to add curls and volume to their straight hair. The approximately six-hour treatment hooked up to what today looks like a torture device would become immensely popular, particularly after World War I. Any woman receiving this permanent wave treatment was susceptible to electric shock and possible hair breakage if she moved while attached to

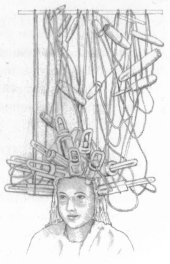

A permanent wave machine from the early 1900s

the waving machine. As my mother said, "All for the price of beauty." Needless to say, Charles Nessler's development was a forerunner of a service that remains popular today.

The Bob Cut

A bobbed hairstyle

Fast-forward to the 1920s and the bob haircut, popularized by Louise Brooks and dancer Irene Castle. In fact, Louise's cut, known as the "Lulu bob," would become an international trend. It heralded a profound change in women's place in the world, for the bob became one of the primary indicators of a woman who knew her own mind and wanted her hair to exhibit this newfound sense of freedom externally. At first, of course, many proclaimed it only a fad; however, it is a classic haircut that endures today and is timeless in its appeal. It brought women in droves into the barbershop, the last bastion of male-dom. Society was aflame with the bob. Men were divorcing their wives, women were threatened with loss of their jobs — indeed, many did lose their jobs. As in earlier historical periods, some spoke out in religious fervor against bobbed women as immoral and disgraceful. Nonetheless, the bob prevailed, and of course the birth of Hollywood, and the sexy screen star, brought a host of new incarnations of the style.

The Flattop

In the meantime the male of the species was in the midst of shipping off to war. The military G.I. Joe flattop, or crew cut as it is still called today, has endured as the bob has endured for women. I remember my father taking my three brothers to the barber when they were little; they all came back with their uniform "buzz" cuts. A bit of wax or pomade would allow the hair to stand up bristly from the top of the head. One thing is certain: This is one of the lowest maintenance haircuts for men to ever arrive on the scene. A major affront to this militaristic and disciplined crew cut came when Elvis Presley burst onto the music scene. What a sensation Elvis would prove to be, not only for his over-the-edge rhythm-and-blues music style, which had not been heard like this before, but also for his entire presence — the heavily pomaded and slicked-back hair, the swiveling hips. Wow!

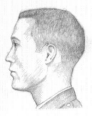

A traditional flattop

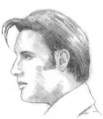

Elvis style

Big Hair

Women in the 1960s would return to a newly stylized version of the 18th-century "big hair." Teasing hair to new heights became the vogue. This required a weekly shampoo and set that was anything but comfortable and, some would say, anything but hygienic, due to the length of time between shampooing and the helmet of hair spray that was needed to get the hair to stay in place. Women carried tail combs on their person at all times in case a sudden scalp itch required relief. Satin pillowcases would keep the style fresh as long as possible.

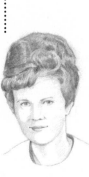

1960s bouffant "big hair"

Peace, Love, and Long Hair

What could possibly come next? Beatlemania! The Beatle invasion in the early 1960s signaled the beginning of a period of great hair turmoil. The long-haired Beatle haircut, coupled with the advent of the Vietnam War and the peace-loving hippie, was pitted against the "Establishment." For both young men and women, long hair was not styled — that

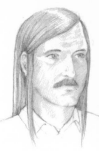

Typical long hairstyle of the 1960s

would be a sign of vanity in a period of war, free love, and finding yourself. Long, straight, and often stringy hair parted down the middle was a symbol of revolt and freedom of expression. Alas, the establishment itself would eventually succumb to the long-hair trend, which even gained respectability among the professional working class. Of course, the professionals visited salon hairdressers and groomed their hair neatly, forgoing the unkempt look that spawned the trend.

The Afro

The 1960s also saw African-Americans allowing their natural hair to grow in and abstaining from relaxing services. The Afro would become a symbol of cultural and ethnic pride; in many cases the style is still worn today for the same reasons.

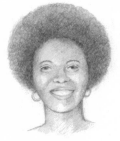

The Afro

The Afro was also considered a natural, healthy way to revive and renew hair that may have been undergoing chemical services for quite some time. Today's hair relaxers, however — when chosen properly for hair type and applied correctly — can serve to condition or manage an overly curly head of hair. I will revisit this subject in a later chapter.

Vidal Sassoon

At about this same time a brilliant hairdresser from London created carefree yet precise haircuts that shocked the world but also came to symbolize women's total emancipation from hair shackledom. Vidal Sassoon's philosophy of not straying from the hair's natural essence in anything that is done to it, from cuts to treatments, coloring, and texture services, was to become the foundation that legions of hair designers stood upon, in turn providing for their clients' wants and needs by adhering to this philosophy. Any haircut performed, Sassoon believed, should honor the integrity of the hair so that the client could experience a wash-and-wear style that would require minimal manipulation. A haircut would become beauty in motion, exuding vitality and a naturally healthy appearance. The hair should have a fluid, liquid feel to it; upon moving, it should fall easily back into the lines of its style. Hair design should accentuate the very best in the individual: her physical appearance, her psyche, and her needs as they related to her lifestyle, right work, and relationships. Vidal has been a mentor to hairstylists from all parts of the globe, and many women today thank him for the revolution he created with his holistic approach to hair and beauty.

Typical Sassoon cut

STYLING IN THE MODERN ERA

A convergence had taken place. Elvis Presley, the Beatles, women's liberation, *Hair,* Vidal Sassoon — they were all important pieces of the mosaic that has brought us into this present era of hair. What crystal ball can tell us how hair will change and evolve around the world in the future? For me the answer lies in one fact, and that is that the herd instinct to following a single fashion is gone. Hair fashion has diversified now into what have been termed "style tribes": a variety of groups, clans, genders, and ages that all create the next statement in style, often simultaneously and around the world.

Living with Popular Culture

Today almost anything seems to go, yet we still look toward other cultures and toward the high-visibility worlds of music, fashion, and sports for fresh ideas. As a society, we often let ourselves be affected profoundly by those of celebrity status as presented in the media, whether in print, on television, or in the film world. Celebrity-watching has become a worldwide phenomenon.

As a hair designer for many years I've had the opportunity to observe society and celebrity. From *The Brady Bunch* to *Dallas* to the newest television serial — images fill our consciousness and can be quite instrumental in creating ideal style in our minds. In a balanced, holistic state, however, you — as the interpreter of your own life — can playfully pick and choose how you would like to present yourself. Have fun and don't take yourself so seriously.

Enjoy popular culture, appreciate its richness, expression, and paradox — it is part of your learning curve in life. As a consciously evolving being, lightheartedness will bring you to a place of great joy while you journey through life. If you want the hairstyle of your favorite Hollywood actress, go for it. Just remember that it is the expression you're re-creating — not who you are. Still, if it is doable, makes you happy, and does not obscure who you are deep down inside, then projecting a certain image or style is quite acceptable.

Expressing Yourself with Style

One thing is certain: We have always and will continue to look for meaning in our hair. This meaning, or feeling or emotion, is connected to the time, place, and culture in which the search takes place. As Professor Steven Zdatny, a modern-day theorist on the political and historical significance of hair, pointed out to me, "The meaning and mood is in the context. The meaning of a Mohawk hairstyle in 1980s London is quite different from a Mohawk in 18th-century New York state."

Your hairstyle is a determining factor in how you look and can tremendously affect how you feel. We all want a style that feels right for us, that captures our essence. This is our individuality, our self-concept — the complex bundle of inherited and acquired traits that comprise our mind, body, and spirit. Our walk and talk, our dress and hair all express who we are below the surface. This is the internal self talking on an external level. This is our personal style.

"The meaning of a Mohawk hairstyle in 1980s London is quite different from a Mohawk in 18th-century New York state."

— Steven Zdatny

And if you feel good in seeing yourself a certain way, if you feel beautiful, vital, and energized, then there is no denying the power of that perception. Self-concept, vitality, and personal style come together to express our individuality.

Every facet of our physicality is a part of our truest nature, as is every thought, emotion, and mood. With that realization, hair can be seen as an important part of who we are. If you are discouraged or unhappy with any part of your appearance, those negative thoughts can manifest in feelings or moods that hinder self-acceptance. One of the premises I'll explore in this book is that our mind, body, and spirit are inextricably linked together. In this sense hair can reflect our state of health — physical, mental, emotional, and spiritual. In its very essence, a natural and healthful approach to beautiful hair can be found in a holistic and nourishing appreciation and care for the vibrant, energetic being that you are. Taking the most nourishing of experiences into our mind-body physiology will go a long way toward building an outward physical expression that reflects the pure and healthful beauty of our spirit.

In addition to whole-body health and an awareness of the products you use, a naturally healthy approach to hair care asks that you recognize the hair virtues that you have and, as the expression goes, "not fight Mother Nature." Wear a style that works in harmony with your hair type, texture, density, and condition as well as your lifestyle. In today's world most of us want freedom from any lengthy styling procedures or large quantities of hair products to make our hair do what we want it to do. No one wants to be controlled by their hair. And this type of freedom can only come from wearing a style that is in total harmony with your nature.

My Own Experience

Growing up on a farm has provided me with a grounding in the natural world, one that came from the food we ate, the organic gardens we grew, as well as my service as caretaker for a wide variety of animals. I fondly remember milking cows, gathering eggs, picking apples, cherries, or pears from the orchard, and spending countless hours in our vegetable and flower gardens pulling weeds. I remember making egg shampoo with my mom, taking a bath in raw milk, and using vinegar or lemon rinses to remove soap. And let's not forget the beer rinse for my hair.

My youth on the farm, the feeling that Nature surrounded and enveloped me in her comforting embrace, was an incredible experience that lives on and is reflected in who I am today. I strive to bring its spirit into every moment of every day, because it was a joyful experience of pure and natural love.

Today, as a wellness consultant, my dharma, or right livelihood — what I'm meant to be doing — is to teach both the conceptual and emotional nature of beauty and wellness integration to cosmetologists, as well as mind-body health courses within my community. It is my desire to share with you this life-affirming knowledge, coupled with what I've learned during a glorious and joyful career spanning 20-plus years. As a beauty educator I've had rich opportunities to travel a great deal and visit a wide variety of countries. This has allowed me to work with all imaginable types of individuals and their hair. Whether in the Mediterranean, Latin America, Asia, Europe, or the U.S., there is one constant to how we feel about hair: It is a very important expression of who we are. It's a part of us.

Hair floats through our dreams and our fantasies. Many see hair as an accessory to be changed at every whim, while others see it as a dear companion and friend to gently nurture and care for while resisting any impulses to change. A change in mood, a change in lifestyle, a trauma, all may be reason to make dramatic changes in hair. Some women are addicted to hair changes like others are addicted to buying clothes. Getting married traditionally inspires the growth of long hair ("for the pictures"), while divorce for many is the time to get a never-before, radical haircut. New hair, new life.

Hair can indeed be an outlet for our very strong desire for self-expression, as well as renewal and reinvention. This is, of course, where things can get pretty darn metaphysical: Finding the right hairstyle for your truest, most excellent self can bring a rebirth, a revival, a renaissance!

CHAPTER 2
The Inside Story: How Hair Grows

Factors that can affect the health of your hair include your age, your general state of health, the environment, and your lifestyle, particularly as it relates to nutrition and exercise. In order to understand how to keep your hair healthy, you need to understand how each of these factors affects hair growth — as well as loss — and nurtures or damages the structure and texture of your hair.

I once read in a medical book that hair can be "a barometer of the soul." By its appearance — its state of health as well as how we style it — hair can indeed mirror what is going on in our minds, and it can also serve as a very good indicator of our general state of health.

TRICHOLOGY

Trichology is the science and study of hair or, more specifically, the science of the physical, emotional, and environmental causes of hair and scalp maladies. The name comes from the Greek word *trichos,* which means "hair." I have taught this subject to many students in cosmetology school.

Cosmetologists have a basic grounding in trichology and are skilled in the art and science of beautifying and improving the hair, skin, and nails, enhancing not only their clients' sense of beauty but also their sense of well-being. Trichologists, on the other hand, have mastered and are certified in trichology based on an extensive amount of training above and beyond their cosmetology licenses. A certified trichologist is the professional to see if you are experiencing problems with your hair

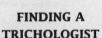

FINDING A TRICHOLOGIST

A trichologist is highly qualified to assess any problems that you may be having with your hair or scalp. The International Association of Trichologists is the best-known organization worldwide for certifying trichologists and can help you locate a trichologist in your area. See Helpful Sources for contact information.

and scalp. Trichologists are very knowledgeable regarding any and all hair and scalp conditions. They will be able to accurately and microscopically examine the hair shaft, the hair bulb embedded in the scalp, and the scalp itself for abnormalities that could be causing certain hair conditions or hair loss.

HAIR COMPOSITION

Hair is 97 percent protein and 3 percent moisture. This strong, fibrous protein, called keratin, also comprises our nails and, in animals, claws, feathers, horns, and fur. What does this mean for you? It points up the two agents that will prove most beneficial in treating hair structure, both internally and externally: protein (to strengthen and fortify) and water, or moisture (to hydrate).

Each hair is an incredibly strong and resilient fiber. However, this fiber has a complex structure that can be easily compromised by all the things we do to our hair — washing, towel-drying, blow-drying, iron curling, chemically changing the color and texture — well, you get the idea. When it's in good condition, a hair is quite elastic; it can stretch up to 30 percent beyond its normal length and spring back. Test your own hair for elasticity by carefully stretching a strand between your thumb and index finger. Release the tension on the strand and see if the hair returns to its normal length. If it doesn't or if it breaks, the hair has poor elasticity. This indicates that your hair is brittle and needs moisture.

Another characteristic to look for in your hair is its *porosity,* or ability to absorb and hold moisture. Healthy hair has the ability to absorb up to 50 percent of its weight in water, and the hair strand can swell up to 120 percent of its normal diameter. Normal hair is porous to varying degrees, ranging from nonporous to slightly porous to extremely porous. When hair is damaged, it loses layers from its protective barrier (called the cuticle — see page 16) and becomes overly porous. To test for porosity, grasp a small section of your hair and rub your thumb and index finger up it, from the ends toward the scalp. If the hair looks excessively rough afterward, it means that your cuticles were standing away from the

HAIR ANALYSIS

Many toxins as well as pharmaceutical drugs that we ingest show up in our hair. One of the more insidious problems in our society is chronic, heavy-metal toxicity, which can lead to a wide range of chronic illnesses. Much of this is the result of environmental contamination, and can have detrimental effects on the brain, kidneys, and immune system. From high aluminum content (linked to Alzheimer's) to lead poisoning, trace and heavy metal hair analysis can uncover some conditions that conventional medical testing cannot. This is carried out by experienced personnel in qualified laboratories.

hair strands and became "frazzled" when rubbed. Another good test — called the sink-or-float test in salons — is to take one hair each from the top, back, and two sides of your head and drop these strands into a bowl of water. If they sink within 5 to 10 seconds, then your hair is overly porous. Such hair is very fragile and should be conditioned thoroughly.

ANATOMY 101

The hair shaft — the part that we see on the outside of the skin — is keratinized, meaning that the soft, collagenous protein growing under the scalp has hardened as it grows outward from the scalp. It is no longer "living," physiologically speaking, and has no blood, nerves, or muscles.

The hair shaft has three distinct layers: the *cuticle,* which is composed of a layer of overlapping cells or scales, like the shingles on a roof; the *cortex,* which comprises the hair's main bulk (up to 90 percent of the hair's molecular weight) and is responsible for the hair's strength, elasticity, and color;

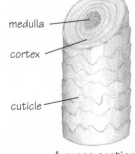

medulla

cortex

cuticle

A cross section of the hair strand

and the *medulla,* a thin core of transparent cells and air spaces often found in the center of the hair strand. The medulla is not always present, often the case in finer hair.

The Cuticle

Think of the cuticle as a coating of armor that protects each hair. The overlapping layers of the cuticle, when lying down and compact, form a tight barrier against repeated assaults from the outside environment as well as from all the mechanical abuse we force on our hair — washing, brushing, blow-drying, chemical changes, and so on. A healthy, compact cuticle also regulates your hair's porosity, acting as a barrier to prevent absorption of excessive moisture

When healthy, the cuticle is translucent and moisturized. Healthy cuticles reflect light, creating a luminous shine and radiance. When the cuticles have been damaged, whether by mechanical, chemical, or environmental stress, the edges of their scales will stand up and away from the hair shaft. This damaged hair will no longer reflect light but instead absorb it, giving the appearance of dull, lackluster hair.

Proper hair care formulas, with moisturizers, proteins, and vitamins, can mend tears and holes in the cuticle while shoring up the vulnerable spots that can allow the inside of the hair shaft to become damaged. However, overprocessing the hair with chemicals or constantly handling it aggressively, such as by rough towel-drying, brushing wet hair, or teasing, can bring hair to the point of no return. Repeated hair abuse can tear chips of cuticle away from the hair shaft, even peeling layers away until there is nothing left but the exposed cortex or core layer. You should never let your hair get to this point — see chapters 6 and 8 for information on preventing or alleviating this type of damage through holistic approaches.

The Cortex

The cortex, which is protected by the cuticle, is where all the vital "stuff" in hair is. This is the powerhouse layer of the hair, where protein and moisture content are substantial.

HAIR TRIVIA

Hair, a primarily nitrogenous substance, is an excellent addition to the compost bin. Nitrogen is a natural fertilizer, a key component of rich, healthy, soils.

Hair is also so absorbent that a hairdresser from Madison, Alabama, has come up with an innovative technique in which hair is used to soak up oil spills. Philip McCrory got the idea while watching the news reports showing the animals affected by the *Exxon Valdez* oil spill in Alaska. He has since patented his idea and NASA is looking at it very closely for its potential applications in space travel. For more information, check out the July/August 1998 issue of *Audubon* magazine.

The cortex is responsible for up to 90 percent of the hair's molecular weight and determines the hair texture. It also houses the pigment, called melanin, that determines your hair color (or the permanent hair coloring you apply to alter the color of your hair).

The cortex layer is made up of millions of parallel fibers of hard proteins held together by a variety of bonds. When these bonds are broken in large numbers and not re-formed, the hair becomes structurally weak. Approximately 80 percent of these bonds are hydrogen bonds, which can be broken by mechanical handling of the hair; approximately 8 percent are disulfide bonds, the strongest bonds in the hair, which can be broken only by chemical means; and the remaining bonds can be broken by some combination of the two. Again, this points to the importance of a vigilant hair care routine that will not compromise the hair.

DESCRIBING TEXTURE

Texture refers to the hair's diameter, which makes for its look and feel — fine, medium, or coarse. When we think of fine hair, we generally think of a more delicate hair structure that feels silky to the touch. Depending on the degree of fineness, this hair can also be described as thin or limp. At the other end of the spectrum we find coarse hair, which has been described as wiry, thick, and full of body. Remember that depending on the condition of the cuticle, fine, medium, and coarse hair can all look shiny and smooth or dull and rough.

The Medulla

This innermost layer, also called the pith, is composed of protein. It is sometimes found in the center of the cortex layer, although it may be absent in fine hair. The medulla has really not shown a function that we need to be concerned about in handling the hair.

THE SCALP-HAIR CONNECTION

The hair and scalp are vastly different yet intricately related. Many times, difficulties with your hair have more to do with the process going on beneath your scalp than with the hair itself. It is directly underneath the scalp's surface that the wonder of hair begins.

An Introduction to Skin

The skin houses the hair. Just as the hair that we see with the eye is made of hardened or keratinized protein, so too a keratinized "dead" layer of cells is seen as the outermost layer of the skin and serves as protection for what is directly beneath the surface. We are constantly shedding surface skin cells as newly keratinizing cells push upward from underneath. This is why protein in our diet is absolutely integral to healthy skin: According to the International Association of Trichologists, about 20 percent of the protein that we ingest is devoted to the skin-replacement process. It is important to mention two points here. First, the outermost visible layer of skin, although "dead," is still permeable to a certain degree; second, when the scalp is not consistently cleansed to remove this layer of dead cells, a buildup of cellular tissue (as well as dried sweat) can result that can choke off the hair follicle as well as create heavy flaking.

Skin is divided into three layers: the *epidermis,* containing the outermost layer of cells; the *dermis,* a substantial layer of tissue underneath the epidermis where the hair growth begins; and the *subcutaneous layer,* a layer of fatty tissue that lies under the dermis and acts as a cushion for the skin.

The Root of the Matter

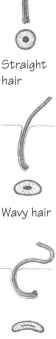

Every hair comes out of the scalp through the hair follicle. The angle at which the hair comes out of the skin is directly related to the shape of the hair. Straight hair is round in cross section and shoots straight out from the scalp. Wavy hair is oval in shape and comes out of the scalp at a slight angle. Curly hair is flattened and comes out of the scalp at an extreme angle.

Straight hair

Each hair has its own blood, nerve, and muscle supply, found within the dermal layer of the skin. At the base of the hair follicle, embedded in the dermis, is the *papilla,* the "root" through which a rich supply of oxygenated blood feeds hair growth via blood capillaries. Blood is the communication link between the body and the hair. Imbalances or toxicity in the body are interpreted and transferred to the hair through the blood supply — or not transferred, as the case may be, such as in a sluggish or blocked flow of blood. Stress, pollutants taken into the body, hormonal fluctuations, illnesses, pharmaceutical or illicit drugs, and poor diet all come into play in this integral part of nourishing hair growth.

Wavy hair

Curly hair

The *hair bulb* envelops the hair papilla. If a hair is pulled out from the root, it is the hair bulb that you see at the end of the strand. Just as a beautiful flower — a tulip, a lily, or a daffodil — sprouts forth and grows from a bulb within rich fertile soil, so too does the hair germinate in and sprout from the hair bulb, growing prolifically with the papilla's rich source of nutrients.

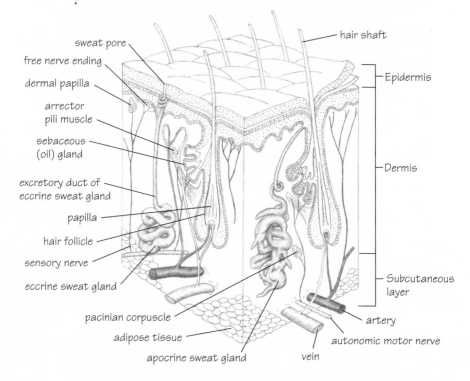

A cross section of the skin allows you to see the different layers and how they function.

DON'T SWEAT IT!

Our hair has its problems — the wind messes it up, the atmosphere does its share, and so do our glands. Glands are found in the dermal layer of the skin. There are two types relevant to a discussion of the hair: sweat glands, which secrete a watery fluid (perspiration), and sebaceous glands, which secrete a fatty substance called sebum.

The Sweat Glands

Secretions from the sweat glands are one of the three ways by which we eliminate toxins from our body (the other two are bowel movements and urination). The body has about two million sweat glands, and they come in two types: the eccrine and the apocrine glands.

Eccrine sweat glands. In the simplest of terms, the eccrine glands are responsible for secreting the sweat that bathes our skin in moisture, maintaining an acid-balanced environment that prevents a proliferation of undesirable bacteria or fungi. We normally excrete 1.7 to 2.6 pints (800 to 1,230 ml) of water during a 24-hour day — but this amount can increase tenfold when we perspire heavily. Perspiration from the eccrine glands also regulates our body temperature by evaporating from the skin, cooling us off when we're overheated. Stress and pungent, spicy foods will also increase the eccrine glands' flow of sweat. Sweat is comprised of water, sodium salts, potassium, sulfuric acid, iron, phosphorus, lactic acid, and urea (a toxic by-product of animal protein metabolism that is processed by the kidneys). The skin will also secrete ingested poisons (heavy metals, arsenic, and so on) if the body's vital functions are all healthy.

Apocrine sweat glands. Body odor is secreted from our apocrine glands, and they are scattered around our body, in our armpits, on our face, chest, and pubic and anal areas. These glands empty into the hair follicles near the skin's surface. Our personal scents change according to our states of health and mind. For example, meat eaters have a smell dramatically different from vegetarians, and a mother can smell the difference in scent between her child and someone else's. Stress can greatly alter the nature of our aroma as well as increase the amount of secretion, because the adrenal glands, when stressed, will increase the output of the male sex hormone androgen (which is responsible for controlling the apocrine glands). The odor is accentuated further by the secretions from the sebaceous glands — sebum — which is a fatty, oily substance that the odors from the apocrine glands cling to. Deposited on the scalp and hair, sebum will absorb odors such as smoke and perfume, as well as any of the more pleasant essential oil fragrances that you may massage into your hair and scalp.

DETOX TEA FOR THE KIDNEYS

Burdock root — whether taken in tincture, capsule, or tea form — is considered one of the strongest blood purifiers in the entire herb kingdom. It is very effective at breaking down and eliminating waste products and tonifying the kidneys. Dandelion enhances the detoxification process and balances the strong cleansing action of the burdock root. Licorice has a slight laxative effect and is quite mucilaginous, coating the digestive tract and stomach lining; it is also a wonderful sweetener and will make the bitterness of the dandelion and burdock root more palatable.

½ tablespoon (8 ml) burdock root
½ tablespoon (8 ml) dandelion root
½ teaspoon (2.5 ml) licorice
1½ cups (375 ml) purified water

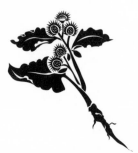

To make:
Place the herbs in the water in a non-aluminum pot and cover. Bring the water to a boil, reduce heat, and simmer, covered, for 5–10 minutes. Strain and discard or compost the spent herbs.

As system maintenance:
Drink 1 cup (250 ml) a day.

As a detoxifying treatment:
Drink 1 cup (250 ml) 3 times a day for 7 to 10 days, and 1 cup a day thereafter. During the first 7 to 10 days, be sure to also drink plenty of fresh water, as this tea is diaphoretic (will induce sweating) and diuretic (will increase urination).

Contraindications:
Licorice is not recommended for use by pregant women, overweight people with edema, or people with high blood pressure.

THE KIDNEYS

Your kidneys are largely responsible for filtering and eliminating toxic waste products from your blood. This is also why, particularly in traditional Chinese medicine, healthy kidneys are equated to healthy hair and skin: detoxification supports a healthy flow of blood and lymph through the body's channels of circulation and makes for dewy, pure, fresh skin and healthy hair growth. To support and nourish the kidneys, drink plenty of purified water every day, minimize animal protein in your diet, eat a whole foods diet, and get plenty of exercise. You can also try the Detox Tea for the Kidneys (facing page), which will work to strengthen and detoxify the blood, kidneys, liver, and gallbladder.

The Sebaceous Glands

The sebaceous glands are the body's built-in automatic lubrication system. There are about 100 per square inch of skin, heavily concentrated on the scalp, face, and upper torso. They are primarily regulated by pituitary-, thyroid-, and sex-gland hormones. They secrete sebum, which serves as a protective mantle for the outer skin and hair and keeps the hair shiny and moist. In puberty the sebaceous glands tend to work overtime, causing skin and hair problems; hair and skin care formulas with astringent qualities will modify and balance such an overabundance of sebum. Conversely, a smooth, consistent secretion of sebum and sweat may be altered and blocked by certain hormonal conditions, age, inadequate diet, and stress. Whether you're experiencing too much or too little sebum, an assessment of your lifestyle and activities, including diet, exercise, and stress, is in order. It is very important to stay the course with gentle, natural, and preferably organic products for the hair and skin. Overcorrecting for oiliness or dryness can exacerbate the problem — many commercial products are nothing other than harsh detergents and pore- and follicle-clogging conditioners. Be guided by your professional hair designer as to the best hair care formulas for your hair and scalp type; if this doesn't remedy a problem with your sebaceous glands, connect with a trichologist or a healthcare practitioner.

WHAT IS HAIR FOR?

Approximately five million hair follicles cover the body. That's right — 5,000,000! The only parts of the body that don't have hair are the lips, palms of the hands, and soles of the feet. Most hairs are very fine, lightly pigmented fibers called *vellus hair.* The remainder — the hair that is darker and visible — is called *terminal hair.* Men tend to have more terminal hair on their bodies because of higher levels of testosterone (the hormone linked to hair growth). Our prehistoric ancestors were covered with terminal hair, but as humans have evolved, the distribution of terminal hair on our bodies has become specific to certain areas.

Hair — here, there, and everywhere — is something that we often take for granted. Yet it is intimately a part of us, both as a part of our external appearance and as a participant in all sorts of physiological machinations going on within.

Protection and Perception

Our scalp hair not only serves an ornamental purpose but also protects the head from the sun; kept covered in cold weather, it prevents body heat — 35 percent of which is lost from the head — from escaping as well. Eyebrows prevent perspiration from running into the eyes, while eyelashes protect the eyes from dust particles. Our nose hairs warm the air that we inhale into our lungs and sweep mucous secretions back down our throat, thus preventing a runny nose.

Our ears also have tiny hairs, located within the fluid-filled inner ear. These hairs move when sound vibrations hit the ear, triggering nerve cells that send electrical impulses to the brain; voilà, we interpret sound! This vibration can also damage our hearing, however, if repeated and loud noise frequencies are constantly assaulting the inner ear.

Insulation

Every single hair on our body is part of a complex insulation system. Attached to each hair under the skin is a muscle called the *arrector pili muscle.* When the skin gets cold, this muscle tugs at the hair, making it stand on end — what we call goosebumps. When this happens, an air pocket forms around the base of the hair that is warmed by the skin.

HAIR GROWTH

Hair is amazing in its prolific growth. In fact, its cell production in the body is second only to that of bone marrow! Our hair grows approximately ½ inch (13 mm) a month, and sometimes slightly faster when we're highly active during the summer months. As we age, however, our hair growth usually slows, and we may even begin to experience hair loss.

Your hair goes through growth cycles. The active growing phase of an individual hair is called the *anagen phase,* and it lasts an average of three to five years. If left uncut, a hair could grow 18 to 30 inches (45 to 75 cm) through this period. The hair then goes into an intermediate or transitional phase called the *catagen phase* just before entering the *telogen phase,* in which it rests for about a hundred days, then falls out. About 85 to 90 percent of all the hair on the head is in an active growing phase at any given moment, while 10 to 15 percent is resting. Every hair follows its own cycle of growth, rest, and falling out, so all hairs grow at different rates. Under normal healthful conditions, you don't need to be concerned that they will all rest and fall out at the same time.

HAIR LOSS

Hair loss, also known as alopecia, is quite common. You can lose approximately 50 to 100 hairs a day and feel fairly confident that this is normal. However, if you experience a steady loss of more than this, it is important to see a trichologist or a medical doctor to have the situation diagnosed. Sudden onset of hair loss can signal other, more serious health conditions and should be discussed with a professional.

Depending on its cause, hair loss may be temporary, such as if it were caused by illness, a dramatic change in diet, or taking or stopping a given medication. Generally this type of hair loss will happen two or three months after its trigger. The body will eventually balance itself, though, and hair growth should return to normal.

Diffuse hair loss, which may occur all over the head or in patches, is not able to correct or balance itself without qualified help. It will be pervasive until its cause — often found to include a hormonal imbalance, mineral deficiency, or anemia — is diagnosed and treated.

Permanent hair loss can result from genetic factors, such as male or female pattern baldness, as well as specific forms of alopecia, especially traction alopecia.

If you're suffering from hair loss or breakage, consider the following as possible causes:

Possible causes of hair loss
◆ Hormonal imbalances
◆ Anemia
◆ Mineral imbalances
◆ Exposure to poisons (heavy metals, pesticides, and so on)
◆ X rays
◆ Many forms of drugs
◆ Liver and kidney disease
◆ Autoimmune disease
◆ Stress
◆ Poor diet, including severe forms of food deprivation such as anorexia nervosa and bulimia
◆ Genetic, hereditary thinning or balding (androgenetic alopecia)

Possible causes of hair breakage
◆ Inherited hair defects (rare)
◆ Fungal infections, such as ringworm
◆ Chemical or mechanical damage or both (from permanent relaxers or waves, or color treatments)
◆ Excessive exposure to sunlight
◆ Poor diet

Possible causes of bald patches

- Alopecia areata (sudden hair loss in round patches), which may be triggered by many factors, including stress, viral or bacterial infection, anemia, and trauma
- Trichotillomania (the pulling out of your own hair)
- Ringworm (a fungal infection)
- Genetic baldness
- Hairstyles worn very tightly over long periods of time, such as braids or ponytails (also known as traction alopecia)

Let me stress that these are only some of the possibilities. I've included this information not so that you might make any form of diagnosis of a hair loss or breakage problem, but rather to make you aware of the wide range of possibilities. If you're faced with hair loss, only a certified trichologist, licensed dermatologist, or your primary care physician can rule out the possibility of a debilitating illness.

JUST THE FACTS

We have anywhere from 90,000 to 140,000 hairs on our head. I don't know that blondes have more fun, but they definitely have more hair. Blondes have approximately 140,000 hairs while brunettes have around 110,000, black hair comes in at around 108,000, and redheads have around 90,000.

Hair Loss and the Endocrine System

The hormonal imbalances that can cause hair loss are related to the endocrine system, that great chemical regulator of the body. Through tiny glands and cell clusters, this system secretes into the bloodstream hormones that control a number of processes, including growth, metabolism, sexual function, and stress response. The endocrine system's effects are slow and relatively long lasting.

The *pituitary gland* at the base of the brain has been called the master gland because the hormones that it produces stimulate other endocrine glands, particularly the thyroid, the adrenal cortex, and the sex glands.

The *thyroid gland* manufactures hormones that regulate the body's metabolism and calcium balance. Calcium is an important nutrient for the hair. An underactive thyroid (hypothyroidism) can cause sluggish metabolism along with a host of other symptoms, including severe hair loss; coarse, dry, brittle hair; and dry, rough skin. An overactive thyroid (hyperthyroidism) can create hair loss as well; it can also create overactive sebaceous glands, hence oily skin and hair. Both of these conditions require medical attention.

The *pancreas* produces insulin to regulate our blood sugar. Blood sugar is what the body uses to fuel its tissues. When insulin levels are too low, hyperglycemia results, or elevated blood-sugar levels. When the insulin levels are too high, hypoglycemia, or lower blood-sugar levels result. Both conditions can create a wide range of symptoms, both physical and emotional, including hair loss. When diagnosed, however, both can be successfully treated. Stress also has a strong effect on levels of blood sugar.

The *adrenal glands* produce many hormones, most notably adrenaline and cortisone, both of which help the body combat stress. An overabundance of these hormones circulating through the system, however, can have very detrimental effects on the hair and skin (see chapter 3 for more details). The adrenals are also responsible for producing a certain amount of androgen (the male sex hormones).

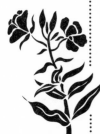

In women, additional androgen production occurs in the *ovaries.* If the ovaries create too much androgen, however, the result is what has been called androgen excess syndrome. (This can also occur if women are on hormone replacement therapies that include too much androgen for their systems.) This syndrome is a common cause of hair loss in women; its symptoms range from mild hair loss to the more extreme male-pattern baldness. This condition can also signal a much deeper problem, from thyroid disease or ovarian cysts to rheumatoid arthritis.

If you are experiencing abnormal hair loss that is not correcting itself, it is imperative to have your hormone levels checked. And if you're overweight, consider this: Excess body fat is a factory for androgen, which — when it's not in balance — can drive up your levels of insulin, as well as blood pressure and lipids.

Living with Hair Loss

Hereditary hair loss in men and women is not related to the hormonal imbalances discussed here. Of course there are many hair regeneratives that may be administered for male-pattern baldness, but I will leave that decision for you to make in consultation with your doctor. These treatments may have to be used on an ongoing basis to maintain any new hair growth; they can be costly and sometimes have side effects.

For both men and women, any hair thinning or loss that's not genetic requires getting at the "root" of the problem, and a positive mind-set is one part of this equation. Hair loss can bring great pyschological distress. It is important to maintain a positive self-image, an appreciation for yourself that goes to the core of your being. It is important to accept yourself unconditionally, and know that you are lovable just the way you are, regardless of the amount of hair on your head. Do notice and have hair and skin issues treated, of course; they can be indicators of disease. But don't become obsessive about your hair if a small amount of thinning occurs. This may be a natural part of the aging process for you. Look after yourself, accept yourself, love yourself, and everything else will fall into place.

DONG QUAI

David Salinger, the executive director of the International Association of Trichologists and an invaluable resource on the subject of trichology, recommends the herbal therapy dong quai for certain women who are having thinning problems. This herb contains substances similar to estrogen (a female sex hormone) and has been shown to influence androgen's effect on the hair, preventing further thinning. It is recommended that dong quai be prescribed by a certified trichologist or herbalist to ensure that it is the right potency.

CHAPTER 3

Healthy from the Inside Out: An Ayurvedic Approach to Hair Care

▼▼▼▼▼

Beautiful hair begins with health — feeling good inside and out. Health (from the Old English *hal,* meaning "whole") is defined as the condition of being of sound body, mind, and spirit. In essence health is a *balance* among these expressions of our being. The body, mind, and spirit are interconnected, and not separate from each other. The spirit, as consciousness, gives rise to the energy and information expressed in our mind and body.

You are the sum of what you think, what you eat, and what you do. Combined, these activities make up your health profile. If you skip meals, eat junk food, smoke, take drugs, drink alcohol, forgo exercise, lack a sense of purpose, are pessimistic, have toxic relationships in your life, and lack spirituality, you are at risk of some form of *dis-ease.* Immune and nervous system malfunctions; hormonal disturbances; heart, lung, and liver disease; and cancer — these are only some of the patterns of disease that may affect us, our health, and in turn our hair and skin.

This subject in itself could fill volumes. However, I will attempt to encapsulate those natural and life-affirming practices that nurture the mind-body physiology and in turn improve the health of your hair (as well as your skin, nails, and teeth). After all, hair is part of you, and the one true premise that unites mind-body approaches toward creating health is that everything — every thought, every action, every atom, and every molecule in our body and in the universe — is connected, and in constant change.

Every day you do one of two things: build health or produce disease in yourself.

— Adelle Davis

AN INTRODUCTION TO AYURVEDA

Ayurveda is a holistic health science that originated in India more than 5,000 years ago. According to Ayurvedic philosophy, true health is simply the result of living a balanced and healthy life, which creates a joyful and vibrant state wherein we are full of energy, creativity, and love. This world tradition is beautifully holistic and accessible to everyone.

The Science of Life

Ayurveda is considered the earliest recorded system developed by humankind to cope with illness. This elaborate system of health is now becoming quite popular in Western civilizations, with thanks in large part going to Deepak Chopra, M.D., a brilliant endocrinologist, healer, teacher, and author who through his teachings is helping societies around the world realize the value of mind-body approaches to health and wellness.

Ayurveda enables you to determine and understand your own unique nature — what is termed in Sanskrit, the classical Indian language, *prakruti* — and it encourages you to maintain a harmonious balance within your nature in every aspect of your daily life. This balance is achieved through meditation, yoga and breathing exercises, the optimal daily routine, nutrition, herbal therapy, massage, and many more everyday practices. All come together to create a profound sense of equilibrium in your life.

Disease is considered a disruption of inner balance — forgetting our memory of wholeness. Ayurveda allows for an acute awareness of states of imbalance in our mind-body physiology, and teaches us how to reckon with them in a healthful and creative way by bringing into action the healing energies inherent in all of us. This elegant system honors our diversity and our individuality, while at the same time recognizing that we are all intimately connected and made from the same "stuff."

> *Every atom belonging to you as well belongs to me.*
>
> — Walt Whitman

Ayurveda and Hair Care

The Ayurvedic approach to health and beauty enhancement is particularly well suited for hair care because in approaching life holistically, you are mindfully creating balance and harmony within your mind-body system. Hair is just one facet that reaps the benefits, yet it is a very pronounced outward expression of your physicality.

According to Ayurveda, beauty is not a stand-alone attribute. Instead, it rests on three pillars: *Outer beauty* includes the appearance of the skin, hair, nails, and teeth; *inner beauty* is the clarity of mind that creates personal confidence; and *lasting beauty* involves the ability to exude health and beauty throughout life.

AYURVEDA AND MODERN SCIENCE

Ayurveda teaches that there are five great elements: space, air, fire, water, and earth. These elements are present in all matter in the universe, including human beings.

- **Space.** This is the expansiveness of the universe that holds the potential for everything — all manifestations of matter come from space.
- **Air.** Air is the element of movement.
- **Fire.** Fire is a transformative power and creates heat, light, and energy.
- **Water.** This is the cohesive element that attracts and holds things together, within our bodies as well as on Earth.
- **Earth.** Any material thing exemplifies earth.

These five basic elements combine in a variety of ways and manifest in the human body as three basic mind-body principles, known as *doshas.* Space and air combine to form the *Vata* or air dosha, that of all forms of movement. Fire and water combine to form the *Pitta* or fire dosha, that of digestion and metabolism. And earth and water combine to form the *Kapha* or earth dosha, the dosha of structure and cohesion.

The lists that follow include thumbnail sketches of the three doshas. All three principles are within each and every one of us, but usually one or two of these forces will dominate. You may have qualities that are equally balanced between two doshas, or you may even be tridoshic, a person in whom all three doshas are of equal value. Your *prakruti* is the dosha (or balance of doshas) that you are born with. *Vakruti* is how your dosha energies may change or be influenced by lifestyle choices. For example, a Vata person, who naturally is filled with movement, can become tremendously unbalanced by lots of additional movement (mental or physical) in his life.

> *The human body is the universe in miniature. That which cannot be found in the body is not to be found in the universe. Hence the philosopher's formula, that the universe within reflects the universe without.*
>
> — Mahatma Gandhi

VATA
Air: "That which moves things"; this is the principle of movement.
Characteristics: Light, cold, dry, irregular, highly active.
Responsible for: All forms of movement of the body, mind, and senses, including thinking, breathing, blood circulation, neuromuscular activity, and gastrointestinal activity.

PITTA
Fire: "That which digests things"; this is the principle of transformation.
Characteristics: Hot, oily, intense, pungent, acidic.
Responsible for: Digestion of food, water, and air throughout the entire system, temperature regulation, energy production, perception, understanding (digestion of ideas, concepts, emotions, and so forth).

KAPHA
Earth: "That which holds things together"; this is the principle of structure and cohesion.
Characteristics: Cold, oily, heavy, stable, slow.
Responsible for: All forms of lubrication, structural creation and stability, holding all the bodily tissues together.

KNOW-YOUR-DOSHA QUESTIONNAIRE

In each category, place a check before **one** or **two** statements that best describe your physical characteristics. At the bottom, add up the total number of check marks in each column. The number of check marks denotes the dominance of each dosha in your unique mind-body constitution, with the column having the most checkmarks being, of course, the most dominant.

Physical Characteristic	VATA (Air)	PITTA (Fire)	KAPHA (Earth)
Frame	❑ I am slender with prominent joints and thin muscles.	❑ I have a medium, symmetrical build with good muscle development.	❑ I have a large, stocky build. My frame is broad, stout, or thick.
Weight	❑ Low; I may forget to eat or have a tendency to lose weight.	❑ Moderate: it is easy for me to gain or lose weight if I put my mind to it.	❑ Heavy; I gain weight easily and have difficulty losing it.
Eyes	❑ I have average or small eyes.	❑ I tend to have an intense gaze.	❑ I have large, pleasant eyes.
Complexion	❑ My skin tends to be dry or thin.	❑ My skin is warm, reddish in color, and prone to irritation.	❑ My skin is thick, moist, and smooth.
Hair	❑ My hair tends to be dry or frizzy.	❑ My hair is fine with a tendency toward early thinning or graying.	❑ I have abundant, thick, and oily hair.
Joints	❑ My joints are thin and prominent, and have a tendency to crack.	❑ My joints are loose and flexible.	❑ My joints are large, well knit, and padded.
Sleep Pattern	❑ I am a light sleeper with a tendency to awaken easily.	❑ I am a moderately sound sleeper, usually needing less than eight hours to feel rested.	❑ My sleep is deep and long. I tend to awaken slowly in the morning.
Body Temperature	❑ My hands and feet are usually cold and I prefer warm environments.	❑ I am usually warm, regardless of the season, and prefer cooler environments.	❑ I am adaptable to most temperatures but do not like cold, wet days.
Temperament	❑ I am lively and enthusiastic by nature. I like to change.	❑ I am purposeful and intense. I like to convince.	❑ I am easy-going and accepting. I like to support.
Under Stress ...	❑ I become anxious or worried.	❑ I become irritable or aggressive.	❑ I become withdrawn or reclusive.
TOTAL	VATA _____	PITTA _____	KAPHA _____

Questionnaire developed by David Simon, M.D., medical director and cofounder of The Chopra Center for Well Being in La Jolla, California (www.chopra.com).

INTERPRETING THE DOSHAS

Can you see in yourself, or others in your life, these qualities and characteristics? The doshas provide a wonderful
understanding of how we can all be so different in our
natures, both physical and mental. Indeed, the doshas can
explain why one person loves a vacation in the Bahamas
while another craves a trip to Alaska, and why one person can
eat incessantly without putting on any weight while another
only has to look at the piece of chocolate cake to put on
pounds. They tell us why one friend may become paranoid,
manic, and highly erratic when out of whack, while another
becomes cynical, obsessive, and jealous, and yet another
becomes aloof, dull, inert, and cloyingly needy. The doshas
can teach us compassion, not only for ourselves but also for
our fellow human beings, because they give us deep understanding. When we come from this place of deep understanding, we become more tolerant and forgiving of those we
are in relationships with when they "push our buttons."

Understanding the doshas, you may begin to understand why your hair or skin may tend to be oily or dry, or
why you may be experiencing diffuse hair fallout or premature graying; you'll be able to learn what you can do in your
daily routine to minimize those things that exacerbate the
problem. Understanding the doshas, you begin to understand and honor your own unique nature, and you see more
readily the signs of upset and imbalance that occur when
you don't honor this unique nature.

At birth the truest expression of our nature, or prakruti,
is expressed in a unique configuration of the three doshas.
This natal dosha configuration can be strongly influenced by
your upbringing, habits, and lifestyle choices. Once you have

> *Understanding how the basic elements of
> nature are expressed in our individual consti-
> tution enables us to make better choices to
> maximize balance and well-being.*
>
> — Deepak Chopra, M.D.

determined your mind-body constitution, you can determine imbalances and go on to pacify and nurture them, bringing the body back into balance. I'm going to explore various approaches to maintaining or restoring a balance — and thus health — within the mind-body physiology. This may seem like a broad approach to hair health, but remember, everything that happens to you is intricately related to every other part of you. Hair that is healthy, systemically speaking, is no more than a reflection of your overall state of wellness.

STRESS MANAGEMENT

The mind is the seat of our emotions, our feelings, our moods. Every thought, feeling, and emotion that we have creates a chemical or molecular reaction in the body that can either enhance or deplete health. Some healers today believe that many of us are disconnected from our deepest, truest selves — what some call the soul — distracted and overwhelmed by the mandates of society: what we should look like, how we should act, who we should be, all as defined from outside ourselves. These healers believe that such loss of self, such psychic fragmentation, is at the root of all stress. Given that we can't separate the emotions from the mind, body, and spirit, Ayurveda gives us a totally natural way to be in a calm, peaceful place where we are more readily able to control stress.

The Stress Response

We now know that stress either causes or exacerbates a large percentage of all disease. Not only heart attacks, strokes, and immune system breakdowns, but almost every disease known has been linked to stressful toxins in our life. How does this link work? Well, stress causes our body to produce toxins, and toxins — those from the food we eat and the environment that surrounds us, as well as those that we produce ourselves when under duress — compromise our well-being. Work-family conflicts, financial pressures, and simply never having enough time are just a few of the many stressors that we face every day.

The biological changes that take place in relation to per-ceived threats are called the *stress response.* Our bodies can adjust for and counteract the mild forms of stress that we encounter. As a matter of fact, stress can be good if we know how to use it to make things happen positively. Pressure can make us face up to challenges with extraordinary skill and fortitude. However, in the case of extreme, unusual, or long-lasting stress — emotional, physical, and chemical — our stress response and the ensuing control mechanisms can be quite overwhelming and harmful. The overflow of stress hormones into our system can adversely affect our mind-body physiology, including our hair and skin.

In prehistoric times, if a caveman out and about doing his hunting came upon a saber-toothed tiger, the alarm and fear that this created would begin the complex reaction called the *fight-or-flight response,* in which adrenaline and other stress-related hormones would begin to surge from his adrenal glands into his bloodstream. This response is designed to counteract perceived danger by setting in motion the body's resources for immediate physical activity. Our caveman's blood pressure would increase, sending blood to his heart, lungs, and extremities; his heart rate would rise; his immune system would be suppressed; his blood's clotting ability would increase. Also, his liver would dump stored glucose into his bloodstream, dramatically increasing blood sugar levels. He'd become superaware and

THE STRESS EPIDEMIC

The World Health Organization describes stress as a "worldwide epidemic." Stress can be defined as "the inability to cope with a threat, real or imagined, to our well-being, which results in a series of responses and adaptations by our minds and bodies." Approximately 80 percent of visits to doctors are related to mind-body stress.

— from The Wellness Councils of America

feel quite strong. Our caveman would now be poised to put up a fight, or run for his life! After surviving this ordeal, he'd have a period of time to recover before being faced with further danger. Having this "downtime" to recoup is the desirable way to handle stress.

Today, our bodies operate the same way. Times of stress produce the same biological and chemical responses, including the production of adrenaline. This adrenaline initially gives the body an energy boost. However, in large or frequent doses, it can also make us feel anxious and nervous. It can create insomnia, depression, fatigue, headaches, digestive upsets, and downright irritability.

It is in facing unrelenting stress, as many of us do these days, that the possibility exists for the stress reaction to keep on humming along even after the fight-or-flight response has worn off. At this stage the adrenals secrete other hormones, such as cortisol and other corticosteroids, that, while necessary when the body is faced with emotional crises, can have very detrimental effects on our health if not controlled. They may increase the risk of a host of significant disease processes, including diabetes, high blood pressure, and cancer. These hormones also have immune system–depressing properties, which can severely compromise the immune system and set up conditions for a continuous string of maladies to take hold, from the common cold to allergies, gastointestinal problems, and much more.

In essence, if we can't manage the stress in our life, we are working our adrenal glands to exhaustion. This is when skin and hair problems also become apparent, because we are constantly shunting our blood supply to our heart and lungs, diverting it away from the feeding and nourishing of the hair, and creating an overabundance of hormones in the bloodstream, overloading the kidneys and creating an internal buildup of toxins.

Learning to Out-Think Stress

The first step toward health comes with becoming aware of all the myriad influences stress has on your mind-body physiology. Given that stress is relative to our *perception* of a given situation, if we are able to change our perception of something or someone, then we are able to change its potential to affect us negatively.

Everyone has a different perception of the same reality. One person could be extremely distraught over an impending divorce, while another feels absolute exhilaration. One individual watching a scary movie might be anxious, with cold, clammy hands and heart beating fast, while another thinks the movie is corny or silly and gets a good laugh from it. Remember, emotions and feelings are all *thoughts.* Recognizing that you have the ability to change your belief, perception, or attitude toward a situation is a powerful first step toward controlling the stressors in your life and creating a harmonious balance.

It is essential to identify, then eliminate or reduce, the sources of stress in your life. Once you have an understanding of your mind-body type, then you can recognize how you deal with stress and try to eliminate negative coping patterns while reinforcing the most positive coping patterns. Some of the most positive health enhancement methods include:

◆ Daily meditation and prayer
◆ Deep breathing
◆ Physical activity including yoga
◆ Optimizing your nutrition

Taking in positive experiences such as these will go a long way toward detoxification on the emotional, physical, and environmental levels.

DEEP BREATHING FOR THE RELAXATION RESPONSE

In view of what stress can do to your health, including the state of your hair and skin, deep breathing is one of the quickest and most reliable ways to achieve well-being. At the same time, deep breathing increases blood circulation to the scalp area, which nourishes your hair. However, although healthy, deep breathing is one of the most natural of acts, a great many of us don't know how to breathe properly.

In Western society we tend toward shallow and rapid chest breathing, or in other words, subtle hyperventilating. Deep breathing creates an internal rhythm that encourages all of the organs and systems in the body to function in physiological harmony. Deep breathing reduces the heart rate, reduces blood pressure, and allows the heart to beat more effectively. It gives a gentle massage to the heart as well as the liver and pancreas, and helps improve the functions of the spleen, stomach, and intestine.

By breathing properly we can learn to relax while controlling our emotions. Energy is increased as more oxygen reaches body cells, thus increasing the metabolism and optimizing nutritional intake from our food. Proper breathing also allows the body to rid itself of the noxious, gaseous by-products of metabolism, especially carbon dioxide.

Practicing Good Breathing

Good healthy breathing depends on the strength of specific muscles. The abdominal muscles must be strong and, more important, so must the diaphragm — the sheet of muscle sandwiched between the lungs and the abdomen. Many people unconsciously hold the diaphragm frozen. The diaphragm should instead push down on the abdomen, expanding it outward with each deep breath into the lungs, then move upward as air is expelled from the lungs.

DIAPHRAGMATIC BREATHING

Go through the following steps and you will be on your way to becoming a better breather:

1. Sit or lie down comfortably, preferably in a quiet place.
2. Place your right hand on your abdomen and your left hand on your chest. Look down and breathe naturally, noting which hand, if either, moves. Ideally, your stomach hand should rise and fall with each inhalation and exhalation, and your chest hand should stay still. (Once you've achieved this, you can leave your hands out of it.)

3. Slowly inhale through your nose so that your stomach hand moves outward. As you breathe in, imagine the warmed air flowing in. Imagine this warmth flowing to all parts of your body.

4. As you slowly exhale through the nose, your abdomen should move inward. As the air flows outward, imagine all of the stress leaving your body.

5. Repeat this process until you achieve a deep sense of relaxation.

You may use this process anywhere, anytime. Many variations exist to heighten the deep-breathing result. You may inhale to a count of 10, and exhale to a count of 10. For quick relaxation, practice deep breathing for a count of 10 breaths. When you have more time, work on this for 10 minutes. If you practice diaphragmatic breathing every day, try to gradually prolong the inhalation and exhalation of your breath. Your body will experience a profoundly deep relaxation and restfulness — more restful than even the deepest sleep. Proper breathing enables you to remain alert and calm simultaneously.

IN AND OUT

When we take in a breath, we breath approximately 10^{22} atoms into our bodies from the environment, and on exhalation breathe out 10^{22} atoms into the environment. This points up just how integrated our bodies are with the environment. In fact, the environment is looked upon in Ayurveda as our extended body.

Pranayama

In Sanskrit, *pranayama* is the science of breath. It is an important part of yoga, which I am going to discuss as well. *Prana* is the life-giving force or energy that infuses us when we use breath awareness techniques, and that brings about the calm, alert sense of total integration among mind, body, and spirit. Remember that the breath is a direct reflection of the mind. The following techniques have very specific results that serve to provide balance for the different mind body types, or doshas.

Try any or all of these breathing techniques to effect profound changes in your mind-body state — physical, emotional, and spiritual. They are superb when used on their own or when you're going into meditation.

ALTERNATE NOSTRIL BREATHING

This technique is called *nadi shodhana*. *Nadi* means "channels of circulation," and *shodhana* means "clearing." Therefore you are clearing the channels of circulation, which helps you center your mind and relieves anxiety or tension. Although great for anyone to do, it is particularly effective for quieting an anxious, overactive Vata mind.

This is a good place to start with this exercise. You may increase the numbers of cycles if desired.

1. Sit in a relaxed, comfortable position with a straight spine.
2. Use your ring finger of your right hand to close off your left nostril. With your mouth closed, inhale smoothly and slowly through your right nostril.
3. Release the left nostril, while closing off the the right nostril with your thumb. Exhale slowly and smoothly out of the left nostril. Breathe diaphragmatically, trying to equalize the lengths of inhalation and exhalation.
4. Repeat this cycle of inhalation through the right nostril and exhalation through the left nostril two more times.
5. Reverse the process of inhalation and exhalation. Inhale through the left nostril and exhale through the right nostril. Do three cycles of breathing this way.

> *Breath is the bridge*
> *which connects life to consciousness,*
> *which unites your body to your thoughts.*
>
> — Thich Naht Hanh

SITALI BREATHING

This breathing technique is very cooling and soothing to the body and therefore excellent for balancing Pitta.

1. Sit comfortably with your spine straight and your eyes closed.

2. Curl your tongue lengthwise to form a tube. The tip of the tongue will protrude from your mouth. Inhale through the mouth.

3. Relaxing the tongue and closing your mouth, exhale fully through your nostrils. Generally the exhale will take slightly longer than the inhale.

4. Repeat six times. Once you're proficient, you can practice this technique for up to two minutes if needed or desired.

Note: If your tongue will not curl lengthwise, roll its tip back to touch your soft palate. Inhale through your closed teeth, and exhale through your nose.

KAPALABHATI BREATHING

Translated, *Kapalabhati* means, "that which makes the head shine." This technique is exhilarating and invigorating. It is wonderful for balancing Kapha. It will stimulate the abdominal muscles and all of the digestive organs. (This technique should not be practiced by pregnant women or individuals with heart conditions.)

1. Sit comfortably with your spine straight and your eyes closed. Place the palms of both hands on your abdomen.

2. Inhale slowly and passively, breathing deeply and diaphragmatically.

3. Vigorously and forcefully exhale through your nostrils, while drawing your stomach tightly inward.

4. Repeat this passive inhalation with forceful exhalation for up to one minute.

This technique provides a quick pick-me-up if you're feeling lethargic or depressed. It has the wonderful effect of massaging the internal organs and the spinal column, increasing the circulation of bodily fluids.

MEDITATION

In 1978, while in Europe on a business trip, I was able to partake of an experience that would be quite transformative and life altering. My cousin Annemieke was managing the Transcendental Meditation Center in Antwerp, Belgium, and was to instruct me over the course of two days in the transcendental meditation (TM) method.

In both TM and primordial sound meditation instruction you receive a mantra, which is looked upon as an instrument of the mind (*man:* "mind," and *tra:* "instrument") that brings you to the deepest and most silent realm of your being. This is described by Deepak Chopra as "going to the silent space between thoughts," a place of infinite possibilities, pure potentiality, pure consciousness, pure spirit. In experiencing this consistently, profound shifts begin to take place in your life — an awakening to the true meaning of existence flows within you. Your mind becomes quite plastic and malleable, so that the little things no longer bother you. "Go with the flow" takes on new meaning.

I stayed with Annemieke for a few days in her flat in Antwerp, and I found her joy in life utterly irresistible. I looked upon her as a being of light who had come into my life at just the right time to serve as one of my teachers. Being brought up in a loving and devoutly Catholic home, I knew what prayer was and understood the value of prayer in caring for the soul. However, meditation was a new concept for me — going into silence to connect with spirit. In a seminar given by Deepak Chopra, a participant in the audience asked Deepak what the difference was between prayer and meditation. He replied, "When you pray you are talking to God, and when in meditation you are listening to God." I found this answer quite profound, and it put many things into perspective for me. Both prayer and meditation allow us to feel the intimate presence of a higher power, and they are both at the heart of our spirituality. Today, as an educator for Dr. Deepak Chopra's organization, Infinite Possibilities Knowledge, I practice primordial sound meditation, and it has brought me greater clarity of mind, enhanced creativity, energy, intuition, and anxiety and stress reduction.

Meditation is a part of virtually all of the world's spiritual traditions, and in it we may find great richness, depth, ritual, and mysticism. In Ayurveda, meditation is the primary practice to use to connect with spirit, to bring balance into your life, and to enhance your health. If you're not in touch with your spirit, your consciousness, then no other modality or health enhancement technique may be of its full value to you.

As Deepak has said, meditation is about "tuning in" and "becoming alert." Meditation has its most profound result when practiced for 20 to 30 minutes twice a day, preferably at dusk and dawn. These are the times in the daily circadian rhythm when a calm and peaceful vibration is most prevalent. Research has shown that meditation slows the heart rate, respiration, and brain waves; in addition, brain wave electrical activity becomes more coherent, muscles relax, and the effects of stress hormones diminish.

Meditation is a practice that will create harmonious balance for all three doshas. It is particularly important for Vatas, to help them quiet their active minds. And it may also be said that we live in highly Vata times — there is a quickening of Vata energy all around us. Meditation is a way to calm and soothe the hyperkinetic world we live in.

MEDITATION PRACTICE

Before going into the stillness of meditation, deep breathing coupled with yoga postures may create a relaxing integration of mind and body. The instructions below will show you how to focus — or rather, unfocus — from the outside world and the incessant chatter going on in your mind by concentrating on your breathing. You may use a personal mantra, such as a chosen word (*peace, love,* or the like) or a chant, or simply concentrate and become aware of your breathing.

1. Sit in a quiet and comfortable place.
2. With your eyes closed, breathe smoothly and naturally, paying attention to the feel of your breath as you exhale, and inhale. Do not attempt to modulate or control your breath in any way. If you feel you are distracted by thoughts, sounds,

or feelings in the body, simply let them come and go as you return your attention to your breath.

3. Continue for 20 to 30 minutes. Then gently open your eyes and bring your awareness back to your surroundings.

4. Practice this twice a day, in the morning and at night.

It is important not to question whether or not you are doing meditation the right way — there is no wrong way. If you find yourself having many thoughts, continue on, because this is a sign that you are releasing a great deal of stress. If you fall asleep this is all right, too; it indicates that you are tired, and your body requires it.

PHYSICAL ACTIVITY

The benefits of physical activity, particularly for the health of our heart and for weight management, are known to all of us. Exercise makes you feel great, and some say it's because chemicals called neurotransmitters, produced in the brain, are stimulated when you exercise. This greatly affects your mood and emotions. Exercise may be the single most reliable way to create energy while at the same time creating relaxation, particularly for women, who tend to have a higher rate of muscular problems from stress. Working up a sweat is great for flushing toxins out of the system, and it also helps to release tension.

The challenge in exercising is to be inspired. You already know it's good for you. Try using your creative visualization skills to propel yourself forward in time, perhaps to see yourself in the "golden" years as healthy, vital, and full of energy instead of bedridden, immobile, overweight, or perhaps chronically ill. Such a visualization experience might inspire you to take the steps necessary to begin or maintain a dedicated physical activity regimen. And make this training something that you look forward to every day because of how good it makes you feel.

Physical activity can be broken down into three different types. It would be great to incorporate a balance of these three types — aerobic, flexibility, and strength-training activities — into your exercise routine.

Aerobics

Aerobic activity pays off in stress reduction, cardiovascular health, and increased immune system function, longevity, endurance, and quality of life. Our bodies are made to move. Metabolic wastes and lactic acid collect internally when we're not moving. Aerobic activities include power yoga, walking, jogging, swimming, biking, cross-country skiing, and dancing. Three 30-minute sessions weekly of aerobic exercise is the recommended minimum. If you're presently sedentary, however, consult with your health care practitioner before beginning. You may need to begin slowly and build to the recommended amount.

Flexibility

This form of exercise involves stretching movements (no bouncing), which will ease physical tension and improve your range of bodily motion and agility; if used as a warm-up or cool-down from aerobics, flexibility exercise may prevent injuries. Flexibility activities include yoga, tai chi, and pilates — all forms of movement that connect your mind and body with their energy source. Try to build stretching movements into your workday, particularly if you stand or sit for long periods of time.

Strength Training

Weight-bearing activities build not only strength but also power and endurance. When you build muscle, you are developing a leaner, fat-burning body. Strength training (including yoga) will also increase your muscle mass and stave off osteoporosis.

Exercise for Balance

Exercise may also serve to balance your dosha type. Vatas benefit greatly from calming, low-impact activities that focus on agility and coordination. Stretching, yoga, brisk walking, bicycling, and dancing are good exercise choices for Vatas.

Pittas, who tend to be competitive, should avoid competitive sports and lean toward moderate activity of all kinds — yoga, jogging, bicycling, hiking, and downhill skiing, to name just a few.

Kaphas, with bodies built for endurance, do well with weight training and vigorous exercise such as power yoga, jogging, swimming, bicycling, cross-country skiing — basically aerobic activity of any kind.

THE ANCIENT ART OF YOGA

Everyone seems to be doing yoga these days, from sports teams to actors to business executives. In Western society, we are most familiar with yoga's fitness component. However, in Ayurveda, yoga is seen as a philosophy of living life with the mind and body intertwined in a mutually supportive relationship; a holistic lifestyle that weaves together fitness, wellness, and consciousness raising.

Yoga has been called "meditation in motion." Concentrating on your breath as you go into yoga postures does indeed have a meditative effect. Regular practice of this invigorating yet calming activity can make you stronger and more flexible while heightening mental awareness.

Yoga is a wonderful activity to perform on its own or as an adjunct to other activities. Yoga can be a complete workout, one that balances every part of you, including the muscles, bones, and breath. Depending on the speed with which you perform yoga and the length of your sessions, it may become an aerobic workout (such is the case is ashtanga yoga, a vigorous, fast-flowing style also known as power yoga). Also, like weight lifting, yoga strengthens your muscles through resistance exercises — except instead of using barbells and machines, you use your body's own weight. Many significant benefits accompany this, including better blood circulation, increased metabolism, improved digestion, enhanced endocrine gland and organ function — the hair and skin become beneficiaries of these enhanced functions.

Classes in yoga are popping up everywhere, from the YMCA to fitness centers. Excellent books and videos are available; see Suggested Reading and Helpful Sources.

A NUTRITIONAL APPROACH TO BEAUTIFUL HAIR

Hair is primarily a transformation of our daily food. Strong, beautiful hair shows that we have a strong digestive system and that we are assimilating our food optimally. Our food choices affect our body chemistry on every level, physical and mental. We can effect great change and bring about balance in mind-body physiology by examining our food choices and making sure we are getting all the nutrients that we need. What could be more simple and beautiful than that?

Eating a balanced diet, preferably of whole foods, will give us tremendous energy; strong, resilient bodies immune to toxins, including stress; and shiny, lustrous hair, glowing skin, and sparkling eyes. According to the surgeon general, 68 percent of disease in the United States is diet related. And 30 percent of cancer is diet related, according to the National Academy of Sciences. Fatigue has become an epidemic, with a primary cause being our intake of highly processed and refined foods — foods that are packed with chemicals while devoid of the nutrients our bodies so desperately need.

Guidelines for a Healthy Diet

Nutrients are the basic components of food, and they satisfy three basic yet vital functions:

- To serve as the fuel that provides energy
- To provide the raw material that renews and repairs body tissues and organs
- To regulate metabolic functions that are constantly occurring in the body

The health of hair and skin depends on the proper supply of nutrients. Taking in foods like refined sugars, certain spices, chemical additives, soft drinks, and so on will be depletive and weakening to the hair, while eating healthy, nutrient-packed foods will give it resilience and strength. The most basic guidelines for good nutrition are:

- Eat a wide variety of foods to optimize nutrients.
- Maintain a healthy weight.

- Choose a diet low in fat, particularly saturated fat, and cholesterol.
- Choose a diet with plenty of vegetables, fruits, and whole grains.
- Use sugars only in moderation.
- Use salt and sodium only in moderation.
- If you drink alcoholic beverages, do so in moderation.

Many thorough books are available on the subject of nutrition, and if you want to create, personalize, or analyze your own diet, you may want to consider consulting with a professional nutritionist.

THE DAMAGE OF DIETING

When entire food groups are sacrificed in pursuit of a svelte body, the hair, skin, and nails pay a hefty price. For example, many people seek to eliminate fat from their diets, when the truth of the matter is that the human body requires a certain amount of the essential fatty acids that comprise fat to carry out vital bodily functions and to absorb fat-soluble vitamins like D, E, and K. The body also requires the calcium, protein, and iron that many dieters give up when they forgo meat and dairy products, as well as vitamin E, which is found in "fatty foods" such as nuts and oils. When the body does not get enough of these nutrients, the hair, skin, and nails are the first to show signs of deficiencies, because the body protects and nourishes the vital organs first — it will conserve its resources to save your kidneys rather than your hair. As a result, hair may become dull, thin, and dry, and you face the possibility of breakage or full-blown hair loss.

If you're going to give up meat or dairy products or both for philosophical reasons, be sure to eat ample amounts of whole grains and beans as well as supplements with flax seed, borage, black currant, or evening primrose oils as alternative sources for EFAs.

There are 40 specific nutrients in our food. These 40 nutrients fall into six categories: carbohydrates, proteins, fats, vitamins, minerals, and water. All of these are part of a healthy diet, but your body needs more of some nutrients than others, depending on your height, weight, level of activity, and, of course, your mind-body constitution.

CARBOHYDRATES

Carbohydrates, found mainly in whole grains, vegetables, and fruits, should account for 55 to 60 percent of our daily intake. Carbohydrates are our body's best source of energy. Through digestion, they are broken down into glucose, which the body uses as energy — the only energy source used by the brain and nervous system. Carhohydrates also supply the fiber our body needs to regulate the digestion, absorption, and circulation of nutrients and regulation of cholesterol levels as well as bowel function — and these functions ensure that the hair is properly supplied with nutrients.

PROTEINS

Proteins are the building blocks of the body and should comprise 10 to 20 percent of your diet. The brain, muscles, skin, hair, and connective tissue are all composed primarily of protein, which we need to produce the enzymes and hormones that regulate body processes. It is important to choose protein sources that are low in cholesterol and saturated fat, such as fish, chicken, legumes, grains, nuts, and seeds.

FATS

Fats supply the body with essential fatty acids (EFAs), which are crucial for many of the body's activities. Fats are also essential for carrying the fat-soluble vitamins into the body. "Good" fats include the polyunsaturated and monounsaturated varieties (which come from plant sources), while "bad" fats are of the saturated varieties (generally from animal sources — meats and dairy — as well as tropical oils like coconut and palm kernel oil). Saturated fats interfere with the removal of cholesterol from the blood. Overall, fat should be approximately 20 to 30 percent of the diet, with saturated fats comprising less than 10 percent of this intake.

OPTIMIZING HAIR GROWTH WITH FATTY ACIDS

For loss, stunted growth, or thinning of hair, Dr. Andrew Weil recommends supplementing the diet with a source of GLA (gamma linolenic acid), a fatty acid that improves the health of hair, skin, and nails. Your choices are evening primrose oil, black currant oil, and borage oil, which are all available in health food stores in capsules. Take one or two 500-mg capsules twice a day. It may take six to eight weeks before you notice a change in your rate of hair loss and thickness of new hair. (As a side benefit, you may also notice that you have healthier, clearer, glowing skin!)

Also try to increase your consumption of omega-3 fatty acids, which have the same positive effects as GLA but also appear to protect against degenerative changes in cells and tissues, by eating more salmon, herring, and mackerel or by supplementing your diet with 1 or 2 tablespoons (15 to 30 ml) of flax seeds (try them ground and sprinkled over food), or 1 tablespoon (15 ml) of flax seed oil.

VITAMINS AND MINERALS

Whole natural foods (of organic origin, if possible) contain the vitamins and minerals that are essential for strong and healthy hair and skin. Without them, our bodies suffer. Vitamin A, for example, is found in abundance in yellow and orange as well as dark leafy vegetables. A deficiency can create a hardened, thick scalp skin that produces a buildup of oil and perspiration below the surface of the skin, with dry hair and flaking dandruff the result. A deficiency of B vitamins, which are so abundant in whole grains, beans, seeds, and vegetables, can create an excessively oily scalp, oily dandruff, baldness, and premature graying. And a nutritional deficiency in the wide range of minerals, which are vital to healthy hair and skin, can adversely affect the structural makeup of the hair as well as the formation of collagen, the connective tissue found in the skin and throughout the body.

We can get all the vitamins and minerals that our bodies require by eating a well-balanced diet and it is preferable to give your body all of its nourishment from a variety of whole, organic foods. However, given the rushed, fast-food mentality of Western culture, many of us don't get these recommended amounts. As a result, many health care providers recommend taking a high-quality vitamin and mineral supplement to make up for any inadequacies of diet and protect our bodies from the assaults of free radicals.

FIGHTING FREE RADICALS

Studies have shown that more than sixty major disorders — and possibly even aging itself — all have the same cause: oxidation, or free radical formation. Free radicals are toxic and highly reactive molecules that are natural products of cell metabolism, and are also produced when the body is exposed to all forms of stress, including mental, physical, and environmental (like solar radiation, X-rays, and pollutants, to name just a few). Free radicals occur when cellular atoms break down, losing electrons in the process. In an attempt to stay balanced, the atom then "borrows" an electron from a neighboring atom, in turn setting up a cascading effect of electron thievery and that ultimately causes the breakdown of molecules, cells, and tissue. Antioxidants reverse the free radical process, establishing order and health on the cellular level, by donating electrons to the imbalanced atoms.

There are many antioxidants, but the most commonly known are vitamins B_6, C, E, beta-carotene (the vegetable source of vitamin A), and selenium. A varied, balanced diet with natural, whole, organic, fresh foods will provide your body with ample antioxidant vitamins; if you're not sure your diet is adequate, try taking a high-quality vitamin and mineral supplement.

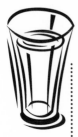

WATER

Water is second only to oxygen as a substance necessary to sustain life. It is the most abundant compound in the body, accounting for approximately 60 to 80 percent of the body's weight. The body needs water to carry out virtually all of its functions, including transporting nutrients throughout the body and removing wastes from the cells. Proper hydration encourages constant, regular elimination, which serves a valuable function in detoxification. Dehydration can create a toxic internal environment and cause a host of bodily malfunctions, including muscle knots and spasms, restricted joint movement, and fluctuating body temperature. Aging is, among other things, a process of drying up. So drink at least eight glasses of spring or purified water daily.

NUTRITION THE AYURVEDIC WAY

In Ayurveda, taste (*rasa* in Sanskrit) is of great importance, as are the temperature and viscosity of food, for creating balance within a given dosha. Ayurveda recognizes six different tastes: sweet, sour, salty, pungent, bitter, and astringent. The inclusion of all six at each meal in the desired proportion for your mind-body type will eliminate the feeling of food cravings that otherwise may lead to overeating and snacking needlessly.

An important element of nutrition the Ayurvedic way is digestion, or the digestive fire (*agni* in Sanskrit), including absorption and elimination. If your digestive fire is not strong, then you won't be able to fully extract the nutrition from the food you eat, creating a buildup of toxic residue (*ama* in Sanskrit) within your body that can greatly hamper its eliminative processes. This makes it very important to eat only when you are sufficiently hungry. You must also learn to eat mindfully, thoroughly chewing each bite of food to begin the digestive process in the mouth. Digestion is then furthered in the stomach, where gastric juices further break down the food into the nutrients to be absorbed through the small intestine into the bloodstream to feed your cells, while the waste is processed for elimination.

THE SWEET TASTE

Description: The sweet taste, composed of earth and water, is basically the taste of sugars and starches, coming primarily from complex carbohydrates, fats, and proteins. This taste has a cooling energy and tends to be oily and heavy. The sweet taste is very nutritive and rejuvenative in nature, promoting the regeneration and building of body tissues. This is a primary taste in the diet for promoting the health and growth of the skin and hair. In excess, however, the sweet taste can cause many disorders, including obesity, diabetes, and lethargy.

Examples: Sugar, fruit juices, honey, rice, whole-wheat bread, whole grains, pasta, milk, cream, butter, ghee (clarified butter), oils, meats, most nuts, sweet fruits (apricots, figs, dates, peaches, melons, pears, and coconut, for example), and vegetables (beets, cucumbers, and potatoes, for example)

Dosha effect: The sweet taste will increase Kapha while decreasing Vata and Pitta.

THE SOUR TASTE

Description: The sour taste, composed of earth and fire, is a fermented or acidic taste. It has a heating energy and is oily and light in nature. The sour taste stimulates the appetite, enhances digestion, and promotes metabolism and circulation. In excess it can cause disorders, including toxic buildup in the blood, excessive thirst, edema, ulcerations, and heartburn.

Examples: Yogurt, cheeses, citrus fruits, green grapes, tomatoes, vinegar, all fermented foods, and pickles

Dosha effect: The sour taste will increase Pitta and Kapha while decreasing Vata.

THE SALTY TASTE

Description: The salty taste, composed of water and fire, comes from mineral salts. This taste has a heating energy and tends to be oily and heavy. It also promotes digestion while increasing the appetite. As a demulcent, salty tastes will soften body tissues. The salty taste is laxative in nature, as well as mildly sedative. Too much of this taste is said to cause graying and fallout of the hair. Some additional

HERBS TO AID DIGESTION

Digestion is the most important part of eating. Nutrients from thoroughly digested foods are absorbed in the intestines and transported through the bloodstream to all the cells of the body, and toxins are eliminated through waste products.

The following are some very effective herbal preparations that can enhance the digestion, absorption, and elimination processes, optimizing the potency of the nutrients you consume:

◆ Fresh, organic gingerroot grated into hot water (to taste) makes for a wonderful tea. Sip on it throughout the day to enhance all of the processes mentioned.

◆ The Ayurvedic preparation Trikatu, a mixture of three pungent herbs, will stimulate digestion when taken before a meal. It's available in most health food stores and from retailers specializing in Ayurvedic products (see Helpful Sources).

◆ The Ayurvedic preparation Triphala, a mixture of three fruits, is a great bowel regulator, specifically to alleviate constipation. It comes in capsule form and is available at most health food stores and from retailers specializing in Ayurvedic products (see Helpful Sources).

disorders could include skin diseases, blood disorders, ulcers, rashes, hypertension, and overheating.
Examples: Sea salt, rock salt, salted nuts, salted fish and meats, seafood, seaweed, kelp
Dosha effect: This taste will increase Pitta and Kapha while decreasing Vata.

THE PUNGENT TASTE
Description: The pungent taste, composed of fire and air, is spicy or acrid and comes primarily from aromatic essential oils. This taste has a heating energy and tends to be dry and

light in nature. It is quite stimulating to the entire physiology — it will promote digestion while increasing the appetite. Pungency will induce sweating, while clearing excess mucus or phlegm from the system. An excess of this taste can cause increased heat and sweating, dizziness, peptic ulcers, and burning sensations in the throat, stomach, and heart.

Examples: All hot peppers (chili, cayenne, and black peppers), ginger, onion, garlic, radishes, mustard, and cloves

Dosha effect: This taste will increase Vata and Pitta while decreasing Kapha.

THE BITTER TASTE

Description: The bitter taste, composed of air and space, is found in alkaloids and glycosides. This taste's energy has a cooling energy and is dry and light in nature. Bitter tastes are anti-inflammatory, antibacterial, and detoxifying. In small amounts, the bitter taste can stimulate the digestion. It also has reducing, depleting, and sedating effects. There is a definite drying effect on the mucous membranes. This can become excessive if too much of the bitter taste is taken. Other disorders could include emaciation, fatigue, and dizziness.

Examples: Bitter greens, rhubarb, turmeric, sprouts, fenugreek, tonic water, and alkaloids like caffeine and nicotine

Dosha effect: This taste will increase Vata while decreasing Pitta and Kapha.

THE ASTRINGENT TASTE

Description: The astringent taste, composed of earth and air, comes from tannins. There is a "puckering" effect from many of these foods. The energy of this taste is cooling and tends toward dryness. The astringent taste is drying, firming, and compacting on the physiology. If taken in excess, it can cause disorders including excessive dryness, constipation, retention of gas, obstructed circulation, and heart pain.

Examples: Unripe bananas, apples, cranberries, pomegranates, broccoli, cabbage, cauliflower, lettuce, spinach, beans, lentils, and tea

Dosha effect: The astringent taste will increase Vata while decreasing Pitta and Kapha.

Guidelines for Your Type

You may wonder how to create a balance of these tastes in your meal, whether you are feeding a family or just yourself. Your best option is to provide a full range of all six tastes and to select from the spread what you know is best for your unique mind-body constitution. For example, if you are of a Kapha constitution, eat more vegetables and smaller portions of bread, rice, pasta, and any animal foods. The reverse holds true for a Vata type — help yourself to more of the sugars (fruits and vegetables) and starches (grains, pastas, rices, and meats) and take lesser portions of bitter or astringent raw salads and vegetables.

It is important that you understand that this brief primer on the six tastes is simply a guide to optimizing nutrition for your mind-body type. Use this information to gauge how you feel. If your food choices give you the energy you require and provide the nutrients your body needs to repair and renew itself, then you can feel confident that you are receiving the optimal nutrition from your food.

Here are some general nutritional guidelines for each of the Ayurvedic types:

VATA
Favor: Oily, warm, and heavy foods that are of the sweet, sour, and salty tastes.
Limit intake of: Pungent, bitter, or astringent tastes.
Avoid: Cold foods and cold drinks; light and raw foods.

PITTA
Favor: Cool or moderately warm foods that are of the sweet, bitter, and astringent tastes.
Limit intake of: Sour, salty, and pungent tastes, as well as hot foods and drinks.

KAPHA
Favor: Light, dry, and warm foods that are of the pungent, bitter, and astringent tastes.
Limit intake of: Sweet, sour, and salty tastes; cold food and drinks, as well as rich desserts.

SYNERGY

It is important to remember that all of the health-giving modalities I am discussing are synergistic in nature. Together, they optimize the flow of energy and vitality. This is the nature of a holistic approach. For example, eating a healthful diet, if done mindlessly or under stress, will prevent you from taking the full amount of nutrients from your food. You need to learn to relax in order to properly digest your food, and many of the techniques I've described here can help you do just that. In turn, physical activity, which can be de-stressing, also enhances the metabolic processes of the food that we take in. All is balance, and finding the routine that is the most natural and life affirming for yourself will bring you to this place.

THREE RULES FOR MINDFUL NUTRITION IN EVERYDAY LIFE

Our Western society is plagued by the dis-ease of obesity. The nutritionally bankrupt yet high-calorie foods that we eat, along with the buildup of toxins in our systems (in the form of partially or improperly digested foods) and our tremendous overconsumption — more than our body needs for its energy expenditure — can not only cause obesity, but more importantly serve as a contributing factor to our high levels of heart disease, cancers, and diabetes.

Remember that eating is a life-affirming act. Eating with awareness and appreciation of the nourishment that you're taking in will increase your assimilation of nutrients. Eat when stressed and your digestive system will function much less efficiently. As you fulfill your biological need to eat with greater awareness and efficiency, you'll reap the benefits: high energy levels and exceptional well-being.

Regardless of the nutritional standards you adhere to — whether it be the USDA food pyramid or Ayurvedic holistic philosophy — if you can follow three general guidelines, you can be sure that you're supplying your body the nutrients it needs for maximum health.

1. As much as you can, eat foods in their whole, natural state. Keep the processing and refinement of foods in your diet to a minimum. Eat vegetables raw or lightly steamed. Snack on fresh, organic fruit. Prepare dishes with whole grains and legumes. Highly processed or refined foods are robbed of nutrients, and their chemical and artificial additives are toxic to our systems. Analyze the ingredient lists of foods that come in a bag, box, or can to determine just how heavily processed they may be. Try to wean yourself off packaged foods, and when you do purchase them, make sure they're made of certified organic ingredients.

2. Choose certified organic foods whenever possible to limit your exposure to chemical pesticides and fertilizers. These chemicals can be very disruptive to the proper functioning of the liver, kidneys, and endocrine and hormonal systems. This philosophy applies to animal products as well — look for the label CERTIFIED ORGANIC and you will be assured that the meat, poultry, or fish was not treated with any form of antibiotics or growth hormones.

3. Eliminate caffeine and concentrated sugars from your diet. This is a tough one for many of us! However, you will bolster your energy levels tremendously by eliminating or radically reducing the amount of caffeine and simple concentrated sugars that you consume. Coffee and other caffeinated beverages are central nervous system stimulants that act on the adrenal glands, causing them to release stored sugar in the liver. The energy that is created will cycle downward, at which point ingestion of more coffee or sweets will cycle the energy back upward. This yo-yo cycling eventually creates adrenal exhaustion.

Overindulging in a cycle of caffeine and sugar consumption tends to sensitize our insulin-producing cells to repeated stimulation. Insulin, as I discussed earlier, is a hormone that helps regulate the amount of sugar delivered to our cells. Frequent sugar consumption can overstimulate insulin activity and remove too much sugar from the blood, creating what is called low blood sugar, or hypoglycemia. This is when tremendous fatigue sets in. The energy highs cycle with fatigue to create an energy roller-coaster ride.

Eating a balanced diet that is natural, whole, and fresh as well as ecologically sound is the primary way to ensure strong, healthy, beautiful hair. Reflect on your eating habits. If you are experiencing problems with your hair or scalp, it just may be that your way of eating is unnatural, extreme, or excessive. Begin a healthy, whole-food eating program and you will see quick and dramatic results in the health of not only your hair and skin but your whole body as well.

A HEALTHFUL SYNTHESIS

Feeling healthy brings with it pleasure and joy. By nurturing your mind, body, and spirit with the techniques I've described in this chapter you will be well on your way to feeling healthy and whole. Remember to approach any and all with an attitude of patience, humility, kindness, and love — toward yourself as well as toward all those you're in relationships with.

The information here is an overview that I hope will inspire you to create your own balancing routine for beauty and wellness incorporating these health-giving modalities. Whether this is the beginning of your journey down a more conscious path toward health, or you have been traveling it for a while, there is enough rich and fruitful information available to you to make this a lifetime journey. And indeed, that is a part of the great joy of life — it is not about the destination, but the journey.

CHAPTER 4

Personalizing Your Hair Care Regimen: Choosing the Right Products

Hair care products are a multibillion-dollar worldwide industry. Whether you're strolling through the aisles of the local drugstore, supermarket, health food store, or your favorite salon, the selection of hair care formulas can be quite confusing, to say the least. There are so many of them! How do you choose the ones that will be best for your hair? My first response to this question is to tell you to rely upon the expertise of a licensed cosmetologist to diagnose and prescribe hair care formulas for your specific hair type, texture, and condition — particularly if you simply do not know how to wade through the plethora of products that line the shelves. Hair designers have received extensive training in how to use the products that are represented in their salons. And I assure you that there are some very good professional products available that will be healthful for your hair.

In the health food store, generally you can be assured that the hair and skin care products available are going to be of a very high quality. In the department or drugstore, your luck will be more hit or miss, of course. You will be reading many labels, trying to decipher what all those ingredients are. And you can be certain that a tremendous amount of time and effort has gone into the marketing, promotion, and packaging of these products, to create a "positioning" in the marketplace that is appealing, that will sell you on the product.

My goal in the following chapter is to give you a primer on what constitutes healthy, natural products for your hair and scalp, as well as what to look for in, and what questions to ask about, some of the not-so-natural chemicals found in many of the commercial products in the marketplace. With this knowledge, you can go on to make intelligent choices as to which products to purchase.

WHAT DO YOU WANT?

According to this top 10 list of desirable attributes, we want products that:

◆ Cleanse without stripping natural oils

◆ Replace lost protein, moisture, and nutrients

◆ Increase and fortify the strength and elasticity of the hair

◆ Protect the hair cuticle

◆ Condition without "weighing down" the hair or building up on the scalp

◆ Even out porosity and prevent moisture loss

◆ Smooth abraded cuticle scales and lock in moisture while creating brilliant shine

◆ Prevent intense drying from the environment through the use of sunscreens

◆ Calm static to prevent flyaway, unmanageable hair

◆ Give an exceptional tactile quality or "feel" to the hair

FROM PLANTS
TO LABORATORIES TO PLANTS

Cosmetic recipes for achieving a more glorious and appealing outward expression of beauty have been found in the oldest recorded literature. Whether by healers, spiritual guides, or cosmeticians, all form of lotions, tinctures, and salves were concocted from natural botanical ingredients; thanks and reverence were given to the spirit of the plant for sharing her special potent powers for transformation and beautification. Plants were harvested according to the cosmic dance found within nature — natural circadian, seasonal, and lunar rhythms greatly influenced how a plant was grown, harvested, and used within a given beauty formulation. Many herbal gardeners today are still strong advocates of this approach, believing that it tremendously enhances the power and intuitive nature of the plant.

At some point the medical and beauty communities made the leap from the natural realm to the synthetic. *Synthetic* refers to formulas produced chemically in a laboratory, rather than being extracted from its natural source. As manufacturing has increased in scale and distribution, storage requirements for beauty products have grown more exacting, as has the desire for an aesthetically "pure," stabilized, emulsified product. Thus the inclusion of all sorts of additives in those original botanicals became the norm. With these additives, large-scale producers attain an extended shelf life for the product without it going rancid or developing bacterial growth; they also achieve a product that has a pleasing viscosity and fragrance without separating. Today, "botanicals" as well as additives may be synthetic in their entirety, or they may include a mix of natural and synthetic ingredients. A select few lines in the marketplace are still of a predominantly natural origin, including Aubrey Organics, Natures Gate, Logona, Geremy Rose, and Weleda, all available through health food stores.

But there are also more and more small companies sprouting up around the country whose philosophy is "less is more." A definite trend is happening here. Through direct marketing, the Internet, and small, specialized "boutique" settings, these companies are teaching a specific and loyal clientele how to buy pure products and personalize them with a variety of herbs, plant and essential oils, and other botanical ingredients. Naturally, they are manufacturing their products using totally natural means.

This groundswell of specialized natural-product companies is creating an impetus for large-scale manufacturers to better their product lines to ensure purity, safety, and healthfulness. Customers are very savvy today, as well as inquisitive about what they are using on their bodies and how it affects both themselves and the earth. There is no doubt about it: We the purchasers of quality hair and skin care products are changing the direction of the industry by demanding pure, natural products.

THE HAIR CARE RITUAL

All of us — men, women, and children — need to cleanse and condition our hair. It is through daily cleansing and conditioning with healthful hair care formulas that we are able to maintain healthy, balanced hair and scalp. The hair can be renewed and refreshed with this regular ritual, and the scalp will shed dead surface skin cells.

Chemicals in many hair products can be harsh, and we're exposed to all forms of pollutants and environmental stresses every day. Depending on your styling routine, you may also be exposing your hair to some treatments and products that are not so healthful. It is for these reasons that your choice of shampoos and conditioners is vital in maintaining your hair in its optimal state.

Shampoos and conditioners are generally classified by the condition of the hair they're intended for. Whether hair is normal, oily, dry, or a combination, the proper choice of shampoo and conditioner can optimize its condition, helping it look naturally healthy and beautiful.

Choosing a Shampoo

There are many types of shampoos. You may see them designated as balancing (for normal scalp and hair), moisturizing (for dry scalp and hair), purifying (for oily scalp and hair), bodifying (for fine hair), or simply for normal-to-dry hair or normal-to-oily hair. Many shampoos claim to contain vitamins and proteins to strengthen the hair. Color-enhancing shampoos have become quite popular, and dandruff treatment shampoos will always be available for those with flaking problems.

Conditioning or 2-in-1 shampoos work well as long as they are not too heavy on the conditioner — some have a very high concentration of conditioner, which ends up weighing down the hair, making it heavy and limp. It all depends on how expertly the shampoo has been formulated. (Do not use this type of shampoo if your hair or scalp is oily.)

A growing trend, particularly in drugstores, is shampoos "for chemically treated hair." In actuality these are shampoos fortified with moisturizers (hydrating), proteins (strengthening), and emollients (smoothing and softening) — all the ingredients usually used for dry hair. They've simply been given a marketing twist by the label FOR PERM-TREATED HAIR or FOR COLOR-TREATED HAIR.

Purifying shampoos — also known as clarifying or alternative shampoos — are used in alternation with your regular shampoo to help prevent the undesirable buildup of minerals (from your water) and to more effectively remove pollutants, styling products, and so on. If you do not use a lot of styling products and wash your hair with softened water, these alternative shampoos should not be necessary.

Choosing a Conditioner

Conditioners come in several varieties. There is the daily rinse-through conditioner that you use in the shower after every shampoo. It works by depositing a coating of positively charged conditioning agents on the hair shaft. This coating remains after rinsing, lubricating the hair shafts and greatly reducing friction, tangles, and knots, thus minimizing stretching of the hair while it is wet and most vulnerable. This conditioner layer also greatly reduces buildup of static and the flyaway hair that results. When properly formulated, this kind of conditioner is good for all types of hair, even fine hair. If a conditioner tends to weigh down your hair, it is creating an undesirable buildup — it may have excessive wax, silicones, or balsam — and is not formulated for your hair type. Switch brands.

Deep protein or moisturizing conditioners (or both) can be used according to your hair's condition. All hair types can use them at least once a month, but it is preferable to apply more often — perhaps once a week — for dry, damaged hair. To apply, leave the conditioner on your hair for anywhere from 5 to 10 minutes while you shower or bathe; or you can shampoo, towel-dry, and then work the conditioner into your hair, cover it with a plastic bag or shower cap, and leave it on for at least 30 minutes before rinsing.

Leave-in conditioners are very popular today to protect the hair from the oxidizing effects from the sun, chlorinated pools, spas, and hot tubs, as well as to protect color-treated hair from fading; they also provide lubrication and protection when you style your hair. To use, first shampoo, use a rinse-through conditioner, towel-dry, and then spray or massage a leave-in conditioner through your hair. This product serves as a good foundation for styling products.

Preshampoo conditioning generally takes the form of hot oil treatments.

READING THE INGREDIENTS LIST

In order to understand what labels are telling you, you first need to understand the rules that govern how manufacturers must provide information.

On retail consumer products, and now most salon products, the ingredients are listed in descending order of predominance (so that the most prevalent ingredient is listed first), down to the 1 percent level. Below 1 percent, ingredients may be listed in any order.

For over-the-counter "drug" products, such as anti-dandruff shampoos, antiperspirants, and fluoride toothpaste, labels must always list first the active ingredient. The remaining ingredients can be listed in descending order of predominance *or* alphabetically.

Remember that many of the products that claim to be natural don't necessarily exclude artificial or synthetic ingredients, even some that are sold in health food stores. Read the ingredients list. And please do remember that both synthetic and natural ingredients have the potential to create allergic reactions.

Following is a short list of some of the categories of ingredients found in hair products, along with their purposes and common ingredients used to perform that function. This is not a complete list. The WorldWatch Institute estimates that as many as 75,000 chemicals are used to make the wide variety of products that most of us use on a day-to-day basis. Many of these can be found in our beauty products.

ANTIOXIDANTS

Antioxidants, as the name implies, provide protection from harmful oxidizing agents which can degrade the quality of hair care products as well as damage your hair and skin. Ozone, chlorine, ultraviolet light, and many environmental pollutants do their mischief by oxidizing molecules to undesirable by-products.

Antioxidants are most often used as food preservatives, protecting their color, taste, and nutritional value. They protect cosmetics in a similar fashion, and more recently their use has been extended to providing protection to the hair and skin. Cosmetic preparations often utilize antioxidants that are natural, such as vitamin A, vitamin C, vitamin E (tocopherol), selenium, zinc, and the amino acid cysteine (extracted from the horsetail plant), as well as antioxidants that are synthetic, such as BHT (butylated hydroxytoluene) and EDTA (trisodium and tetrasodium edetate).

ANTISEPTICS

Antiseptics destroy or inhibit the growth of the scalp microorganisms that can cause problems such as dandruff. Herbs, as natural antiseptics, are preferable to harsher synthetic varieties. Strong antiseptic herbs include aloe, burdock, chamomile, rosemary, and sage. Tea tree essential oil is also a strong antiseptic.

CARRYING AGENTS

Carrying agents are used as the base of a preparation; they "carry" the active ingredients. Herbal extracts (also called "teas") should preferably use water, vegetable glycerin, or grain alcohol as their carrying agent, not propylene glycol.

CHELATORS

Chelators are purifiers that bind impurities firmly to themselves, then rinse down the drain. Citric acid, which is found widely in plants, is preferable to synthetic chelates.

DETERGENTS

Detergents are synthetic soaps made from a variety of chemicals. They are used in shampoos for their cleansing properties.

They do their work by emulsifying oils and suspending dirt particles on the scalp and hair, to be rinsed away. Many detergents used in shampoos can be harsh and potentially allergenic, including sodium lauryl sulfate and NDELA (nitrosodiethanolamine) that's formed with TEA, DEA, or MEA. These ingredients are on the FDA list of suspected carcinogens. Some manufacturers use a harsh detergent then add buffers to lower its pH (a measure of acidity or alkalinity). Many of these are not biodegradable — check the label!

EMOLLIENTS

Emollients inhibit the loss of moisture and thus have a softening, smoothing effect on the skin, scalp, and hair. They're excellent for dry, damaged, or difficult-to-control hair. All forms of vegetable oils provide natural emollience.

Synthetic emollients include mineral oil (which can contain carcinogens) and silicones. Also be aware that synthetics with PEG-n designations *may* contain 1,4-dioxane, a carcinogenic ingredient that is a manufacturing by-product. Fatty alcohols like cetyl and cetearyl alcohol have been shown to cause contact eczema in certain individuals. And esters like cetearyl, isopropyl, polyethylene, propylene, and stearyl alcohols (to name only a few) have been shown to cause allergies and dermatitis.

EMULSIFIERS

Emulsifiers are added to a product formulation to hold together opposites like oil and water, creating a uniformly blended consistency. Mayonnaise is a good example of an emulsion. Lecithin is one of the most effective natural emulsifiers. It is made up of a variety of phospholipids (by-products

▼▼▼

CONSUMER POWER

Essentially you have two choices: You can create your own hair care formulas, or you must carefully select a hair care treatment regimen from what exists in the marketplace. Both options require that you become as informed as you possibly can about ingredients, but the latter involves self-education in labeling practices. By becoming informed purchasers of personal care and hair care products, we drive manufacturers to evolve and create the most healthful and effective products possible, while eliminating harmful substances from the marketplace.

▲▲▲

of soybean oil manufacture, as well as poultry eggs). Phospholipids also serve as natural humectants. Synthetic emulsifiers include any alkoxylated alcohols; all compounds with MEA, DEA, TEA, and MIPA; and all ingredients with the prefix PEG-n or PEG. All may be potentially carcinogenic given the possibility of nitrosamine contamination.

FRAGRANCE

In natural preparations, essential oils are used for fragrance. If the ingredients label simply lists "fragrance," with no further identification, chances are it's a synthetic ingredient. Synthetic fragrances have proven to be the most prevalent sensitizer (cause of allergic reactions or chemical sensitivities) in cosmetic preparations.

HUMECTANTS

Humectants are used to attract, hold, and retain moisture, optimizing the hair's resilience, suppleness, and elasticity. Through their moisture-absorbing properties, they give hair body and a feeling of fullness. Humectants also prevent products from drying out. Natural humectants include vegetable glycerin and sorbitol. The most prevalent synthetic humectants include propylene glycol, butylene glycol, ethylene glycol, and PEG or polyethelene glycol (according to FDA, highly allergenic). Propylene glycol is popular because it's very effective, but it causes irritation and contact dermatitis in many users. A synthetic humectant that is quite safe and effective is isosteroyl lactylate.

LUBRICANTS

Lubricants reduce friction between hair strands while smoothing the hair and adding shine. They are beneficial because of their protective qualities. Silicones and plant oils are widely used to provide lubrication.

MOISTURIZERS

When used externally on the hair or skin, moisturizers raise moisture content, rehydrating dry hair and scalp while restoring flexibility. A wide range of natural moisturizers exist; they include amino acids, aloe vera, evening primrose oil, panthenol, olive oil, and lanolin. There are also many of the synthetic variety including cetyl alcohol, dimethicone silicone, isopropyl lanolate, myristate, and palmitate.

PRESERVATIVES

Preservatives give hair care products an extended shelf life (usually three years) by preventing product deterioration. They are also antimicrobial in nature. Natural preservatives include wheat germ and vitamin E oils, as well as citric acid. Some of the common synthetic preservatives that are potential allergenics are the parabens, quaternium-15, and imidazolidinyl urea. (See also Antioxidants on page 68.)

PROTEINS

Proteins can substantially strengthen the hair shaft by bonding to and filling damaged sites within it. The proteins of choice are from the vegetable world: wheat and soy protein. (Milk protein is also a preferred source.) Synthesized proteins are quite effective and when hydrolyzed can be of a molecular size that will be quite substantive in the hair. There is no reported toxicity for synthesized proteins.

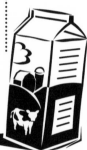

SILICONES

Silicones are complex compounds that are emollient and lubricating in nature, providing a high water and temperature resistance that enhances flexibility, protection, and light-reflecting shine. These compounds should be used sparingly for the best results, because in excess they can create a buildup, weighing the hair down. (See also Lubricants on page 70.)

SUNSCREENS

Hair is just as prone to sun damage as the skin and scalp are, particularly in today's ozone-depleted atmosphere. The sun is a powerful energy source that will oxidize the pigment in hair and damage the hair shaft. Sunscreens (such as benzophenone-4) protect the hair from some of this damage; they can also provide a measure of protection to the scalp. If your hair is thinning, however, or if you're partially bald, you'll also need to apply a sunscreen for the skin.

SURFACTANTS

Surfactants lower the surface tension between the many ingredients found in cleansing formulas, allowing the product to spread more easily. Surfactants occur naturally in plants like soapwort, yucca, and quillaya. Natural soaps — made from vegetable sources like coconut oil, palm kernel oil, or olive oil — are surfactants, and so are synthetic detergents.

Synthetic detergents include PEG-8 (polyethylene glycol), which is on the FDA's list of suspected carcinogens. And any compounds that include DEA, MEA, TEA, or MIPA may form nitrosamines, which have been determined to cause cancer.

Some newer synthetic surfactants are made from natural fatty acids and sugar, or from simple amino acids. These can be a good choice, as they are nontoxic, biodegradable, and very gentle. On the label these will appear as sucrose, polyglucose, or glutamate.

VITAMINS

Vitamins are absorbed into various levels of the hair shaft to provide emollient (smoothing) properties as well as antioxidant and shine-enhancing capabilities. Panthenol, or vitamin B_5, is an ingredient in many shampoos and conditioners. It has been proven substantive to the hair, thickening and strengthening it while adding shine.

INGREDIENTS TO BE WARY OF

Hair care products contain many synthetics and petrochemicals that have been proven allergenic, and perhaps even toxic. The FDA considers many of these ingredients safe because the amounts used — particularly in shampoos — are purportedly low enough to do no harm, and the product itself is intended to be thoroughly rinsed from the hair, having only brief contact with the skin. However, research has simply not determined what the long-term adverse reactions to these synthetics are, not to mention what effects the manufacturing of these chemicals, and washing them down the drain, might have on Mother Earth.

With the large amount of chemicals that we are all exposed to day in and day out, multiple chemical sensitivities are becoming epidemic in our society. If you use shampoos or conditioners that contain synthetic chemicals, it becomes even more important to thoroughly rinse them out of your hair, to ensure that no residual chemicals are left on your scalp.

The ingredients outlined here are the most pervasive in hair care products. Studying this list should provide you with a starting point to evaluate labels as you shop.

COCAMIDE DEA, MEA, OR MIPA

These are synthetic surfactants used in soaps and many shampoos. They are often referred to as natural and "derived from coconuts." In high concentrations they can be allergenic; they may also be contaminated with nitrosamines, a potent class of carcinogens. If you choose to use any products that contain nitrosamine-forming agents, make sure that vitamins A and C are also in the products; these serve as blocking agents.

IMIDAZOLIDINYL UREA AND DIAZOLIDINYL UREA

These commonly used preservatives are also antiseptic and deodorizing. They have been established by the American Academy of Dermatology to be primary causes of contact dermatitis (causing adverse reactions such as rashes that can be quite severe). Keep clear of the sensitive eye area.

THE PARABENS

These preservatives, including methyl, propyl, butyl, and ethyl parabens, inhibit microbial growth and extend a product's shelf life. They are known to be allergenic. Note that parabens are also used in processed foodstuffs. You can eliminate the parabens altogether and opt for natural alternatives: vitamins A (retinyl), C, and E (tocopherol); essential oils such as sweet orange, peppermint, or rosemary; or citrus seed extracts like grapefruit seed oil. *Note:* Food-grade parabens are used in personal care products in very low quantities — but this does not change the fact that they have been proven highly allergenic for certain individuals.

PROPYLENE GLYCOL

This is a petroleum-derived humectant, surfactant, solvent, and carrier that is known to cause allergic reactions. It will show up in the ingredients lists of many "natural" products, and again is found in many items that we ingest, including ice cream, bakery goods, children's cough syrup, and mouthwash. As a humectant, the natural alternative is vegetable glycerin, a natural, syrupy alcohol used as a lubricating base for cosmetics.

SODIUM LAURYL SULFATE

This widely used synthetic detergent and emulsifier has been proven to cause eye irritations, skin rashes, hair loss, and allergic reactions. The label may say that this ingredient is derived from coconut. Sodium lauryl sulfate has been linked to nitrosamine formation. Opt for the gentler cleansing action of sodium laureth sulfate or one of the new state-of-the-art surfactants now available — particularly the alkyl polyglucoside class of gentle surfactants, which show great compatibility with the skin and hair. The raw ingredients used to create alkyl polyglucosides are sucrose, glucose, and fatty acids. These are fully biodegradeable and have no reported side effects.

Note: In 1983, a panel of independent physicians and scientists assembled by the Cosmetic, Toiletry, and Fragrance Association deemed sodium lauryl sulfate safe as long as it's washed off quickly and thoroughly — the way shampoo is.

READING THE LABELS

Following are some sample ingredient lists of hair care products in the marketplace. Study the ingredients and their positioning. Remember, the lists are arranged in descending order of amount.

"BALANCING" SHAMPOO FOR ALL HAIR TYPES

Highly synthesized product ingredients list: Purified water, sodium laureth sulfate, ammonium laureth sulfate, lauramide DEA, cocamidopropyl betaine, dipropylene glycol, citric acid, hydroxypropyl methylcellulose, tetrasodium EDTA, sodium chloride, DMDM hydantoin, glycerin, sodium lauryl sulfate, propylene glycol, cocamide DEA, glycol stearate, cetyl palmitate, benzophenone-4, panthenyl hydroxypropyl steardimonium chloride, tocopheryl acetate, lauryl polyglucose, wheat germamidopropyldimonium hydroxpropyl, hydrolyzed wheat protein, fragrance, FD&C yellow no. 5, FD&C yellow no. 6.

Highly "herbalized" product ingredients list: Coconut oil, olive oil castile, vegetable protein (soya), water, Roman chamomile oil, rosemary, sage, nettles, coltsfoot, horsetail, aloe, vitamins A, C, and E, panthenol, Inositol, niacin, preserved with citrus seed extract.

DAILY RINSE-OUT CONDITIONER
FOR ALL HAIR TYPES

Highly synthesized product ingredients list: Purified water, cetyl alcohol, cyclomethicone, stearyl actyldimonium methosulfate, stearyl alcohol, nonoxynol-10, glycerin, tallowtrimonium chloride, hydroxyethylcellulose, citric acid, stearamidopropyl dimethylamine, methylchloro-isothiazolinone, DMDM hydantoin, disodium EDTA, methylisothiazolinone, sodium PCA, hydrolyzed soy protein, hydrolyzed wheat protein, panthenyl hydroxypropyl, steardimonium chloride, benzophenone-4, fragrance, tocopheryl acetate, retinyl palmitate.

Highly "herbalized" product ingredient list: Water, extracts of chamomile, nettles, ho-lien-hua, nelumbo nucifera, comfrey root, cherry bark, schleichera trijuga, kusambi bark, burdock, and yucca, vegetable emulsifying wax, coconut oil, methylparaben, oil of myrrh, oil of lavender.

The Bad News

If you read the lists carefully, you'll note that several ingredients in the highly synthesized products are not "healthy,"
they even seem downright alarming.

- **Benzophenone-4.** May cause severe contact dermati-
  tis in some individuals, as well as photosensitivity.
- **Cetyl alcohol.** May cause contact eczema.
- **Cocamide DEA.** Nitrosamines, which are carcino-
  genic, can form in this class of chemicals.
- **Cocamidopropyl betaine.** May cause eyelid
  dermatitis.
- **Dipropylene glycol.** A form of propylene glycol.
- **Disodium EDTA.** Carcinogenic nitrosamines can
  form in this class of chemical.
- **DMDM hydantoin.** May cause dermatitis.
- **Fragrance.** May cause contact dermatitis.
- **Glycol stearate.** Can cause delayed contact allergies
  and other adverse reactions.
- **Lauramide DEA.** Nitrosamines, which are carcino-
  genic, can form in this ingredient.
- **Methylchloroisothiazolinone.** May cause allergies.
- **Methylisothiazolinone.** May cause allergies.
- **Propylene glycol.** Causes delayed contact allergies,
  skin irritation, and dermatitis in some individuals.
- **Sodium lauryl sulfate.** This detergent can be very
  drying to the hair and skin. It is also a proven aller-
  gen and skin irritant.
- **Stearamidopropyl dimethylamine.** Belongs to
  amines group, which may cause allergic dermatitis
  and have carcinogenic properties.
- **Stearyl alcohol.** May cause contact dermatitis and
  allergies.
- **Tallowtrimonium chloride.** A quaternary ammonium compound. All quaternary ammonium compounds can be toxic, depending on the dose and
  concentration. A skin, eye, and mucous membrane
  irritant.
- **Tetrasodium EDTA.** Nitrosamines, known carcino-
  gins, may form in this class of chemicals.

Study the differences. The highly synthesized and chemicalized formulas are enough to take your breath away!

Note that *some of the ingredients listed here are considered favorable synthetic ingredients with no known or recorded toxicity.* But how benign is that chemical when applied topically to the body and flushed down the drain into the earth? What about its biodegradability? Chamomile can create skin irritation in certain individuals, but it comes from the earth, and to the earth it returns when rinsed from the hair and skin. Synthesized versions of chamomile may not interact so harmoniously with our bodies or our planet. Synthetic wheat protein or natural wheat protein? Natural coconut oil or a synthesized oil? Natural glycerin or a synthesized version? I don't mean to oversimplify this issue. Just remember that the choices you make will have an impact on your health and, ultimately, on the health of the earth.

ASSESSING YOUR HAIR AND SCALP

FOR NORMAL TO DRY HAIR, FOR NORMAL TO OILY HAIR, FOR FINE HAIR, FOR REMOISTURIZING, FOR DEEP PROTEIN CONDITIONING TREATMENT, FOR BODY BUILDING, FOR THICKER HAIR . . . these are just a few of the descriptions you'll find on the labels of shampoos and conditioners. There are as many different categories of shampoos as there are conditioners. That is why it is important to know your hair quantity, type, diameter, texture, and condition in order to select wisely from the many products on the shelves.

The *quantity* or *density* of your hair is the number of hairs per square inch on your head. This information is not necessary to select shampoos and conditioners, but it can determine how long you need to rinse your hair after these treatments in order to remove all residue; thin hair will not need to be rinsed as long as thick hair. And density will be of utmost importance in determining the style that you are going to wear.

There are generally four hair *types:* normal, oily, dry, and chemically treated (chemically treated and dry hair types are often the same), as well as combinations of these. These categories are useful when considered along with the hair *diameter,* which can be fine, medium, or coarse, and hair *shape* or *texture,* which may be straight (round), wavy (oval), curly (flattened), or a combination (erratic mix). These categorizations are helpful, although it is important to note that a wide range of subtle variations exists.

It is important to note here that virtually any *condition* of the hair and scalp may be assessed, and a course of treatment prescribed to correct, balance, or maintain a given condition. Your professional cosmetologist can be invaluable in helping diagnose your hair and scalp condition. It is also important to see a professional trichologist, dermatologist, or other healthcare provider if there is any indication that a hair or scalp condition may be other then externally influenced.

Assessing Your Hair Condition

Hair can be oily and dry at the same time, and so can the scalp. The hair and scalp are in fact always changing — according to the seasons, according to hormonal fluctuations, according to changes in lifestyle or nutrition, and so on. If your hair is color treated, you could have dry, damaged ends and an oily scalp. In a case like this — as in any instance where there are dramatic differences between hair and scalp conditions — you'll need to strike a balance, treating the oily scalp without accentuating the dry hair condition.

Normal hair. We all would like to say our hair is normal. The word *normal,* however, is a specific term used to describe hair that is strong, resilient, moisturized, and shiny — whether fine, medium, or coarse in diameter, and straight, wavy, or curly in its shape or textural movement. A normal scalp is one that is moist and pink without any form of irritation, redness or bumps (these may be symptoms of folliculitis, an irritation of the hair follicles). The goal with normal hair and scalp is to maintain this balanced state.

Oily hair. Oily hair is not very prevalent today because of the amount of shampooing that we do, which keeps excess sebum at bay. Oily hair usually means oily scalp. Fine hair tends to take on a limp, greasy look if the sebaceous glands are working overtime. Adolescents often experience this condition; the hormones do balance and normalize over time, though, given a healthy diet and lifestyle. In all cases of oily scalp it is important to choose a gentle cleansing shampoo that will wash away excess oil without exacerbating the problem. It is very possible that you will need to select a shampoo for an oily scalp while choosing a conditioner for dry hair lengths.

Dry hair. Dry hair is dull, lackluster, and, at the extreme, brittle in its appearance. This type of hair feels hard, not soft and silky. It craves moisture, and in most instances requires a healthy dose of protein. Dry hair needs protection in the form of emollients and lubricants, which will lay down the outside cuticle layer of the hair and create shine. Humectants will attract and retain moisture within this type of hair.

Hair may be dry for a variety of reasons. This may be a natural condition of the hair, especially with very curly or frizzy hair. Dryness can also be created by the products used on the hair — shampoos, styling products, and the like. It can occur after mechanical treatment of the hair, such as styling or chemically treating with color, waves, or relaxers, or as a response to environmental conditions like sun, chlorine, salt water, or forced heat in cold climates. A dry scalp can be created by harsh products used on the hair, or by not thoroughly rinsing products out of the hair and off the scalp. Many people who think they have dandruff don't have dandruff at all — they simply have a flaking scalp from a buildup of dry cells, mixed with shampoo and conditioner residue that has not been thoroughly rinsed from the hair. A thorough massaging of the scalp during each shampoo is absolutely necessary to remove this buildup. Hormonal and environmental conditions can certainly create as well as aggravate a dry scalp. And a dry scalp can be an internally created condition, as discussed in chapter 3, if your diet does not include enough of the essential fatty acids and vitamins to maintain moisturized, lubricated skin. Shampoos and conditioners chosen for dry hair and scalp conditions need to be quite nutritive in nature to smooth the hair and build its strength, while adding moisture.

Combinations. Following are some of the more common hair and scalp combinations. I give these as a guide to help you assess your own hair and scalp types and then select wisely from the hair care products available. Remember that normal, oily, or dry conditions may occur on fine, medium, and coarse hair types. It's all relative.

- **Normal scalp and hair.** It is desirable to maintain this balanced healthy state with a regular daily cleansing and conditioning routine.
- **Oily scalp and hair.** Try not to overstimulate the scalp with aggressive manipulations or products, so as not to create extra sebum production. Gently cleanse every day. Try to minimize the amount of styling products you use.
- **Dry scalp and hair.** Daily cleansing and conditioning with moisturizing and emollient treatments will go a long way toward alleviating a dry, tight scalp, while replenishing lost moisture and proteins along the hair shaft.
- **Oily scalp and dry hair.** Gently cleanse every day with a cleanser for normal to oily hair types. Another option you'll find is a balancing shampoo for normal hair. Alternate this at least once a week with a purifying shampoo (also called a clarifying shampoo). Apply a moisturizing conditioner of any type specifically to your dry hair areas.
- **Oily scalp and normal hair.** Treat the oily scalp condition as outlined above while using a conditioner throughout the lengths of hair.
- **Dry scalp and normal hair.** Use rich, nourishing shampoos that are moisturizing on the scalp. Generally these will be designated as shampoos for dry hair or for normal to dry hair types.

EIGHT STEPS
TO THE PERFECT SHAMPOO

Now that you know more about the hair care products out there, let's turn to the actual experience of shampooing and conditioning the hair. Most of us go through this process without giving much thought to it. The following guidelines, however, can make it the most pleasurable and healthful experience possible.

Remember, regular shampooing followed by a conditioner or rinse will give your hair more moisture and shine. Shampooing also gives your scalp muscles and hair follicles a stimulating boost, which in turn can encourage healthier hair growth.

Step 1. Wet the hair thoroughly with warm water. Do not wash or rinse your hair with hot water; it is as drying to the hair and scalp as it is to the skin.

Step 2. Put a small amount of the shampoo in the palms of your hands and spread it by rubbing your palms together. Touch your palms gently onto different areas of your head to distribute the shampoo. Now begin the shampoo manipulations and massage. Work from the front hairline above the eyebrows toward the crown area using small circular movements. Take your time! Work from the side hairline toward the center back of the head with the same movements. Finally, work through the nape area. Use the pads of your fingers to manipulate your scalp. Lift your fingertips and move them slightly each time instead of dragging them across the scalp. Concentrate on moving the scalp as you shampoo. If you have longer hair, whisk your hands down and through your hair at intervals throughout the shampoo to distribute and cleanse the lengths of hair. A shampoo should minimally last two minutes; with longer hair it could take three minutes.

Step 3. Rinse, rinse, and rinse again. This step is crucial to remove all residue, particularly from shampoos that contain a motherlode of synthetic chemicals. Massage the hair gently as you rinse, lifting it away from the scalp if you have long or thick hair, and then let the water flow back and through your hair as you stand under the showerhead.

QUICK TIPS FOR SHAMPOOING

- When shampooing and rinsing, always work from the scalp area out to the ends. This is the direction of the cuticle scales.

- Try not to cluster or bunch longer lengths of hair as you massage; this can cause tangling.

- Don't vigorously rub the hair against itself while you shampoo or condition. This will roughen and stress the hair shaft, particularly the cuticle scales.

Step 4. Don't apply commercial conditioners directly on your scalp unless they specifically instruct you to do so. You want to use these products on the hair where they're needed. Depending on the length of your hair, work a small amount into your hands and apply as needed, to dry ends or through the entire length of your hair. Lightly massage or stroke through the strands. Then rinse thoroughly as instructed in step 3.

Step 5. Very gently squeeze or blot your hair dry with a highly absorbent towel. Never tousle, twist, or wring your hair with a towel or your hands; friction can erode the cuticle. This is a key to healthy hair. The more moisture you can remove in the towel-drying process, the less you'll need to use a blow dryer.

Step 6. Apply the desired leave-in conditioner appropriate for your hair type.

Step 7. Use a large or wide-toothed comb to comb out your towel-dried hair. If your hair is long, begin with the underneath sections, then work up to the top of your head. Separate or finger-comb your hair when possible. Avoid brushing wet hair to detangle it and avoid metal combs, as they can snap or break the hair.

Step 8. Apply the desired styling products, then style.

DEALING WITH DANDRUFF

Pityriasis or dandruff is an inflammation of the skin characterized by abnormal formation and flaking of skin cells from the scalp. If you have dandruff, you will generally know about it because of the excessive flaking in the hair that shows up on your collar and shoulders. Dandruff is in fact a symptom, not a condition, and can arise for a number of different reasons. There has been some debate as to what causes dandruff. However, the majority of dermatologists believe the cause to be a fungal yeast known as pityrosporum. Dandruff may show up as dry and white scales (pityriasis capitis), or yellowish, oily flakes or scales (pityriasis steatoides).

Antidandruff shampoos in the marketplace can be fairly harsh. Keep in mind that these should be used for only a limited amount of time to control the situation. If they don't bring your dandruff under control, you'll need to see a trichologist or dermatologist for further treatment. Evaluate the many fine options for dandruff treatment that are available in the health food store, and see chapter 6 for some homegrown treatments.

Dandruff can be a symptom of the following conditions:

- **Seborrheic dermatitis** is a red, scaly, itchy rash that creates either dry or greasy scaling not only on the scalp but also on the face. The scalp will respond to regular brushing (to loosen flakes), as well as to receiving olive oil massages.

- **Cradle cap** is a seborrheic condition in infants that's harmless if the scalp does not become infected. Cradle cap is characterized by thick, yellow scales on the infant's scalp. This condition tends to recur. Mild cradle cap is best treated with a mild shampoo designed to treat the problem. Olive oil can also be gently rubbed into the baby's scalp and left overnight to loosen the scales before brushing and cleansing.

- **Neurodermatitis** is a stress-related condition that resembles psoriasis. It appears as a single intensely itchy patch with small dry scales.

- **Psoriasis** is a common recurring skin disorder sometimes triggered by stress and hormonal changes or infection. With psoriasis, new skin cells are formed 10 times faster than normal, resulting in well-defined red patches of flaking, silvery scales that can be quite itchy. Psoriasis is best diagnosed and treated by a healthcare provider.

- **Contact dermatitis** is a flaky, itchy, and sometimes blistered rash formed in reaction to some substance coming in contact with the skin — often the chemicals found in color, wave, and relaxer treatments, as well as shampoos, conditioners, and styling products. Sometimes small blisters will appear, rupturing and forming crusts. In later stages, if the irritant has been continuously applied, the skin will dry and thicken and scales will appear as the cells accelerate their rate of replacement. It is imperative with contact dermatitis to determine what the irritant is and eliminate it. When this is done, the condition should clear up within a few days. If the condition persists or is severe, it is important to consult with a trichologist or dermatologist.

A FINAL REMINDER

Treat hair as gently as possible. Remember that hair is a fiber. And just as you provide the gentlest treatment to your finest washables, so you should take this same approach with your hair. Treat it like a fine silk blouse, not a pair of denim jeans, and you will be able to appreciate luxurious, silky, and shiny hair. I have been amazed at how some people treat their hair and then wonder why it looks so bad! There is a lot of ugly, dry, brittle hair walking around out there on the streets, and this does not have to be the case. When your professional cosmetologist educates you as to what he or she is using, why, and how, ask whatever questions you need to understand how to keep your hair looking beautiful and healthy every day. It does not have to be a high-maintenance routine, but it should take into account the styling products and procedures you use — letting them work in synergy with your holistic approach toward your hair and overall health.

CHAPTER 5
Using Ingredients from Nature
▼▼▼▼▼

You will find many of the ingredients discussed here in your garden, kitchen cupboards, refrigerator, local health food store, or nearby apothecary — as well as from the suppliers listed in Helpful Sources. The most delicious part about all of this is that these ingredients are born of the earth. This makes for a very magical and powerful experience. The spirits of the plant impart their vibrational energy, their potency, into hair and skin care formulas, just as the energy and information that we take in through our food renews and vitalizes our body. Every single living species is interconnected, and our love of and reliance on the plant world is irrevocable. We become the plants that we eat. So, too, do our hair and skin reflect the nurturing that we provide them with ingredients from the natural world, whether in products we purchase or those we make.

Let's look at some of the ingredients we can use to create our own hair care formulas.

PLANT OILS

These oils are extracted from fruits, vegetables, grains, nuts, or seeds. Used for their emollient, moisturizing, and lubricating qualities, for both skin and hair, they're also called base or carrier oils, because they're used to dilute essential oils, and to create herbal oils by the addition of herbs. These oils can also be used by themselves for their soothing, nutritive properties — particularly for massage. Make sure to use pure, organic oils; they will say PURE COLD-PRESSED or PURE EXPELLER-PRESSED on the label.

Note: Do not use mineral oil. It is petroleum based and very harsh on the skin, with no nutritive benefits whatsoever.

ALMOND
Also called sweet almond oil, this light, odorless oil is rich in protein, vitamins, and minerals. This mild oil is good for all skin types and has an excellent shelf life.

CANOLA

This lightweight oil comes from the the Canadian grapeseed plant. It is readily absorbed by the skin, although it does have less nutritive value than some of the other oils. It serves as an excellent base for essential oils. It can be used on all skin types and is odorless and high in oleic acid, which resists rancidity.

CASTOR

From the pressed seeds of the castor plant, this oil has excellent emollient, lubricating, and absorbing qualities. A high level of fatty acids make this oil quite soothing to the skin and hair. Its thicker viscosity is excellent for Vata constitutions.

COCONUT

From the fruit of the coconut palm tree, this emollient oil has a cooling quality and is therefore good for sensitive, inflamed skin conditions. It has very large molecules, so absorption into the skin and hair is minimized. It has been used often in folk medicine as a hair conditioning and moisturizing oil.

JOJOBA

From the beanlike seed of the desert shrub jojoba, this oil is technically a liquid wax. It has excellent softening and moisturizing qualities, particularly for the scalp and hair, because it so closely emulates the natural sebum from the scalp. It is lightweight, highly emollient, and contains nutrients that feed the skin. Easily absorbed, it is a great carrier for essential oils and herbal extractions.

OLIVE

From the fruit of the olive tree, this cooling oil is rich in protein, minerals, and vitamins. It will impart a rich, nongreasy emollience and shine to the hair. It nourishes, stimulates, and softens the skin. The vitamin E in olive oil is a powerful antioxidant, and the fatty acids make for an oil that is very stable (it resists going rancid). This oil is heavier in viscosity and has a stronger aroma than most other oils, so, depending on your personal preference, you may want to mix it with a lighter oil. Make sure to purchase the "extra-virgin" variety. This cooling oil is preferred by Pitta types.

SAFFLOWER

This oil comes from the seeds of a thistlelike composite herb. A lightweight oil, it contains proteins, minerals, and vitamins and can be used on all skin types. Safflower oil has one of the highest linoleic acid contents of all known oils. This fatty acid compound gives the oil superior compatibility with the skin and excellent moisturizing capabilities, because the moisture content of the skin is proportionate to its essential fatty acid content.

SESAME

This is one of my favorite all-purpose oils. Made from sesame seeds, it is a very nutritive oil, high in vitamins, minerals, proteins, lecithin, and amino acids. The high level of phytosteroids (sterolins) in sesame oil make this an excellent moisturizer and conditioner, and its high level of antioxidants make it very stable. It also has natural sunscreen properties. Recent studies have shown that sesame oil, which contains high levels of linoleic (fatty) acid, has antibacterial, antifungal, and anti-inflammatory properties, and may play a role in halting the growth of cancer cells.

SUNFLOWER

From the seeds of the beautiful sunflower, this emollient oil, containing nutritive vitamins and minerals, may be used on all skin types.

VITAMIN E

This oil is an excellent antioxidant, or free radical scavenger, and thus a superb preservative. This vitamin can penetrate the skin completely.

WHEAT GERM

Wheat germ oil is also an excellent antioxidant and preservative. It is rich in vitamins A, B, C, D, and E — in fact, it has the highest vitamin E content of any oil. It also has high levels of fatty acids and lecithin. Both vitamin E and wheat germ oils are excellent when added (in small amounts) to your plant oil preparations.

HERBS

By now, most of us can relate healing experiences that we have had with herbs — echinacea to build the immune system, ginseng to manage stress, ginkgo biloba for memory, saw palmetto for prostate health, ginger for nausea — the list goes on and on. Herbs are also common ingredients in cosmetic preparations — henna for tinting, comfrey for soothing, horsetail for strengthening, chamomile for emolliency, and many more. Ancient wisdom and folkloric methods have been the starting point for exploring herb usage, and of course today the scientific community looks to quantify everything it can about herbs. They're no longer an alternative therapy — they're good medicine!

The following herbs have proven efficacious for the hair and scalp. This is the short list, of course; many others exist.

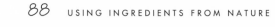

ALOE VERA *(ALOE VERA)*
The gel found within the leaves of this plant has remarkable properties, including healing, soothing, antibacterial, antiseptic, emollient, and moisturizing qualities. Studies have shown aloe enhances cellular regeneration. The juice from aloe vera has been used as a shampoo, hair setting lotion, and conditioner, with remarkable results for both the hair and the scalp. Diseases of the scalp are often treated directly with aloe vera juice.

BASIL *(OCIMUM BASILICUM)*
This aromatic herb, a member of the mint family, is soothing, purifying, and stimulating. It is an effective hair conditioner and detangler. Claims have been made that it is a hair growth stimulant.

BAY LEAF *(LAURUS NOBILIS)*
This wonderfully aromatic herb adds a warming quality to any preparation. It is antiseptic, soothing, and stimulating.

BHRINGARAJ *(ECLIPTA ALBA)*
In Ayurveda, this herb has been called "the ruler of the hair," because it promotes hair growth. Used in a medicated oil, it

is said to be famous for making the hair luxurious, and reversing graying, hair loss, and thinning. It is tonic, rejuvenative, and anti-inflammatory.

BURDOCK *(ARCTIUM LAPPA)*
When taken internally as either a decoction or tincture, this plant is a powerful blood cleanser. Burdock is astringent and regulates sebum. It is also antibacterial, antiseptic, and anti-dandruff. Mineral rich, the stimulating oil extracts from the root and aboveground plant are quite smoothing to the skin, and promote hair growth.

CALENDULA *(CALENDULA OFFICINALIS)*
Also called marigold, this healing plant has stimulating, anti-inflammatory, and demulcent (mucilaginous) properties. Good for sensitive skin, it also promotes the healing of skin tissue. It is an emollient that has softening and soothing effects on the hair and scalp.

CHAMOMILE *(CHAMAEMELUM NOBILE, MATRICARIA RECUTITA)*
Extracts from this flowering herb are used in preparations for sensitive skin because of its sedative and emollient effects. The active principle in chamomile is alpha-bisabolol, which is anti-inflammatory, antimicrobial, antiseptic, and nonallergenic. Also used in hair dyes, chamomile has a brightening and shine-enhancing quality, particularly for blond hair.

COLTSFOOT *(TUSSILAGO FARFARA)*
This herb is excellent for the hair. It is valued for its high levels of amino acids (cysteine), phytosterols, and silica. This herb is said to strengthen, condition, and make the hair more resilient — thickening hair strands and enhancing shine. It's also a great normalizer for excess oil production of skin and hair.

HENNA *(LAWSONIA SPP.)*
Henna leaves are used as a coloring agent, and the plant in its entirety has wonderful conditioning properties. It is important to buy pure henna that does not contain metallic salts; these can create a buildup on the hair that may prove damaging.

HERBAL PREPARATIONS

When you work with herbs, make sure that they are as fresh as possible, or use good-quality dried herbs, infusions, or tinctures. Here are some general guidelines:

Dried or fresh? If a recipe calls for dried herbs, you can substitute fresh herbs by tripling the amount called for. If a recipe calls for fresh herbs, you can substitute dried herbs by using one-third the amount called for.

Infusions. Herbal teas generally made from leaves and flowers. Pour boiling water over the herbs, cover, steep for at least 20 minutes, and strain. Use 2 tablespoons (30 ml) of dried herbs for every cup (235 ml) of water.

Decoctions. Herbal teas generally made from fibrous parts of plants, such as roots, branches, or seeds. Place the herbs in water, cover, bring to a boil, let simmer for up to 10 minutes, then strain. Use 2 tablespoons (30 ml) of dried herbs for every cup (235 ml) of water.

Tinctures. Potent herbal extracts formulated by steeping the herbs in alcohol, vinegar, or vegetable glycerin. Place 2 parts finely chopped fresh herb in 5 parts diluted grain alcohol (mixed in a 1:1 solution with distilled water), vinegar, or vegetable glycerin base in a glass container. Seal, and let steep for up to a month, gently turning the jar every day or two. Strain the tincture through a cheesecloth into dark glass bottles, seal tight, and store in a cool, dark location. Tinctures can also be purchased at health food stores and herb shops.

Herbal oils. "Herbalized" or infused oils can be prepared by either steeping the herbs in a base oil for several weeks, or mixing an herbal decoction with oil and simmering it until all the water has dissipated from the mixture.

HORSETAIL *(EQUISETUM ARVENSE)*

This herb is excellent for the hair. Like coltsfoot, it's valued for its high levels of amino acids, phytosterols, and silica and is said to strengthen, condition, make the hair more resilient, and normalize oil production of skin and hair.

LAVENDER *(LAVANDULA OFFICINALIS)*

The flowering tops of this herb have a delightful aroma. Lavender has cleansing and astringent qualities. It is also very beneficial as a cellular regenerator for the skin.

LEMONGRASS *(CYMBOPOGON CITRATUS)*

This herb has antioxidant, astringent, and freshening qualities for the hair. It is very effective in cleansers and as an oil regulator — it is said to enhance fullness, body (particularly in fine hair), and shine. The lemony aroma makes a wonderful addition to hair care preparations.

MARSH MALLOW *(ALTHEA OFFICINALIS)*

Anti-inflammatory and astringent, marsh mallow is said to both control oil production and soothe allergic or inflammatory skin conditions. The mucilaginous nature of the herb makes for its emollience. It's good for sensitive skin.

MINT *(MENTHA SPP.)*

Wonderfully fragrant, mint is refreshing, stimulating, and invigorating. It is antiseptic and anesthetic in nature, creating a cooling, soothing effect.

NETTLE *(URTICA DIOICA)*

Nettles contains mucilage, amino acids, minerals, vitamins, and other beneficial herbal constituents that make this a very nourishing herb. Nettle is tonic (strengthening) and antifungal; it's also said to stimulate circulation at the scalp, which is beneficial for hair growth. If you're gathering it in the wild or garden, be sure to harvest before it flowers, and wear gloves so you're not stung by the glandular hairs along its stalk. Interestingly enough, the burning and irritation caused by nettle plant hairs may be alleviated by dabbing nettle tea on the skin.

OREGANO *(ORIGANUM VULGARE)*

This aromatic herb is stimulating, antiseptic, and astringent (having good cleansing properties). Oregano is effective as a hair detangler and softener.

PARSLEY *(PETROSELINUM CRISPUM)*

This aromatic herb from the carrot family is high in fatty acids, vitamins, and minerals. Antimicrobial and tonic, it is healing, cleansing, and soothing. When rubbed on the scalp, parsley oil purportedly stimulates hair growth.

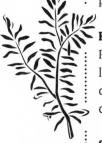

ROSEMARY *(ROSMARINUS OFFICINALIS)*

Purifying, antimicrobial, antiseptic, astringent, and stimulating, this aromatic member of the mint family is a tremendous conditioner for the hair. It can also be used at higher quantities in a rinse to darken the hair.

SAGE *(SALVIA OFFICINALIS)*

This fragrant herb is purifying, antimicrobial, cleansing, and astringent. Like rosemary, it is a tremendous conditioner for the hair.

SOAPWORT *(SAPONARIA OFFICINALIS)*

This perennial herb, a native of Europe, creates a lather in water when agitated. Its active principle is saponin, a detergent that can be a good substitute for soap, especially when making shampoo formulas.

THYME *(THYMUS VULGARIS)*

This aromatic herb is stimulating, antimicrobial, and antiseptic. It has an equalizing effect on oily skin.

ESSENTIAL OILS

Whether you're peeling an orange, planting your face in a bouquet of roses, or crushing mint leaves, the aroma that wafts to the olfactory bulb in your nasal cavity will send its mood-altering effects to your brain. Any essential oil, whether extracted from trees, herbs, flowers, roots, or fruits, has hundreds of powerful chemical constituents that act on our bodies either physiologically or psychologically. The therapeutic and mood-enhancing qualities of essential oils are undeniable — and extensive studies have borne this out.

Whether we inhale the gaseous vapor of essential oils that have been released into the air or apply them to the body externally, the essential oil molecules are absorbed into the bloodstream. This is the oil's single most important property: when used externally, the molecules are small enough to penetrate the skin, reaching the dermis layer and interacting with sensory nerves, blood vessels, lymph vessels, hair follicles, and the sebaceous and sweat glands. Essential oils have a proven ability to promote elimination of waste matter and dead cells while increasing the regeneration of cells. In hair and scalp preparations, the nutrients and proteins in essential oils, as well as their circulation-stimulating properties, oxygenate the blood, which in turn greatly enhances cellular activity and regeneration and gives hair the nourishment it needs for rich, healthful growth.

Essential oils vary greatly in cost and quality. Your health and whole food store will carry a supply of pure essential oils or should be able to order them for you. You can also order directly from essential oil companies (see Helpful Sources). Strive to purchase organically produced oils.

BASIL

This spicy scent is also sweet and very refreshing. It has excellent cleansing, antiseptic, and toning properties. It's especially good for oilier conditions.

Contraindication: Basil may be too stimulating for use during pregnancy.

THE PATCH TEST

Whether using herbs, herbal formulas, essential oils, or commercial preparations, be sure to first do a patch test to test for possible allergic reactions.

Apply a small amount of the preparation either to the area inside your elbow, or directly behind your ear. If over the next 24 hours you experience any redness, itching, or burning — or if a rash forms — do not use that particular preparation.

BERGAMOT

The essence from a citrus fruit, this sweet and fruity fragrant oil is astringent, antiseptic, and deodorizing. Use it for normal to oily scalp and hair conditions; it is also helpful in dandruff and seborrheic conditions.

CARROT SEED

This fragrant, soothing oil is especially useful on dry scalp and hair conditions. With its high vitamin B and A content, it also works as a sunscreen.

CEDARWOOD

This spicy fragrance has stimulating, antiseptic, astringent, and soothing properties that make it valuable for a variety of skin and scalp conditions. It is said to be beneficial for hair loss and thinning, as well as dandruff and psoriasis.

CAUTIONS

If you are going to work with essential oils, I strongly suggest that you educate yourself about usage guidelines. Essential oils are concentrated and volatile, and they can be harmful if used improperly. **Do not take essential oils internally, except under the advice of a knowledgeable healthcare provider.** Except for some of the milder essential oils, such as lavender, most essential oils need to be diluted in a carrier oil before being applied.

Some essential oils shouldn't be used during pregnancy or when health problems exist. During the first three months of pregnancy, consult your healthcare professional before using any essential oil. Also note carefully any specific contraindications mentioned with each essential oil. And keep all essential oils away from your eyes and away from children.

Remember to perform a patch test (see page 93) before using any of these essential oils on your skin.

CHAMOMILE

The fruity, warm Roman variety and the sweet, herbaceous, and fruity blue chamomile both have similar characteristics: They are anti-inflammatory, antiallergenic, antiseptic, and astringent. Chamomile is exceptional in treating dry, sensitive, or inflamed skin.

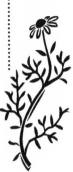

CLARY SAGE

This cleansing and refreshing oil may be used for normal as well as combination skins. It has a vitalizing action on the scalp. It is excellent for dry and mature skin, regulates dandruff and seborrheic conditions, and preserves moisture in the skin.

Contraindications: Clary sage may be overly sedating for those with low blood pressure.

CYPRESS

The sweet and balsamic aroma of this oil brings you to the depths of a pine forest. Astringent and antiseptic, cypress is very soothing for sensitive skin types and effective on dandruff and psoriasis conditions as well as an oily scalp or hair.

Contraindications: Cypress may be too stimulating for use during pregnancy.

EUCALYPTUS

With its powerful fragrance and strong camphor note, eucalyptus is antiseptic, antibacterial, and stimulating (cool), yet sedative in nature. It is very useful for an oily scalp or hair.

GERANIUM

This powerful oil is richly sweet and rosy, with fruity and minty undertones. It has anti-inflammatory, antiseptic, astringent, and stimulating properties. It equalizes oily conditions of the scalp and hair. Given its intensity, use a quarter to half the amount you'd use of other oils.

JASMINE

This oil is very uplifting, stimulating the brain and inducing euphoria. This very expensive essential oil has an intensely floral, warm, and rich aroma with herbaceous, fruity undertones. Use it for normal and combination conditions; also, with its antiseptic, toning, and anti-inflammatory properties, it is well suited to skin that is dry or sensitive as well as to dermatitis conditions.

JUNIPER

This stimulating oil has a clean, fresh aroma that is warm, balsamic, woody, and sweet. Antiseptic, astringent, and anti-inflammatory, it has a cleansing, toning effect on the skin. It is good for normal as well as oily scalp and hair conditions, and it's also effective for dandruff and dermatitis.

LAVENDER

This wonderfully therapeutic and calming oil has an aroma that is sweet, balsamic, and herbaceous, with floral, woody undertones. This oil stimulates while relaxing. It's adaptogenic in nature, meaning that it normalizes both dry and oily conditions of the scalp or hair — in essence all types. Antimicrobial, anti-inflammatory, and skin regenerative, it is also great for sensitive or mature skin, and dandruff, inflammatory, and hair loss conditions.

Contraindications: Lavender may be overly sedating for those with low blood pressure.

LEMON

From the peels of ripe lemon, this oil has a fruity, clean, fresh, and invigorating aroma. Antiseptic, astringent, antibacterial, cleansing, and cell regenerative, it is useful on all skin types, but it's exceptional in regulating sebum production for an oily scalp or hair. It is also used on blond hair for its brightening, shine-enhancing capabilities, and is effective for inflamed skin and dandruff conditions.

LEMONGRASS

Warm and woody yet fresh and lemony, this aromatic oil is distilled from the leaves of the plant. It has antiseptic, astringent, and stimulating properties. It is also effective against fungal infections. This oil is powerful and can cause allergic responses, so use it in small amounts.

MARJORAM

This warming oil is very calming. It features a sweet herbaceous aroma. Softening and soothing, this oil is well suited to sensitive scalps.

NEROLI

From the flowers of the bitter orange tree, this oil is floral, light, and refreshing. It has anti-inflammatory and skin regenerative properties. Quite calming, it is good for normal, combination, dry, and mature skins.

ORANGE

Sweet orange oil is sweet, fruity, light, and fresh. Calming yet stimulating, this oil is emollient, astringent, toning, and antibacterial. It is well suited to oily skin with its toning properties, yet also good for dry, sensitive, and mature skins because of its regenerative properties.

PEPPERMINT

Strong, fresh, sweet, and minty, this oil also has balsamic undertones. It's cooling, cleansing, stimulating, and invigorating. Antiseptic, toning, and anti-inflammatory, this purifying oil is well suited for oily, inflammatory, dermatitis, and dandruff conditions.

Contraindications: Peppermint should be used with caution by those who have high blood pressure, as it can raise the blood pressure.

ROSE

This very costly oil is astringent, toning, antiseptic, anti-inflammatory, and skin regenerative. The warm, deeply floral aroma is slightly spicy with nuances of honey. This oil can be used on all skin types, but it's excellent for sensitive, inflamed, dry, and mature skin.

ROSEMARY

This oil's invigorating and woody, herbaceous odor has camphor undertones. This is one of the most dynamic oils for hair care. It improves circulation and is antiseptic, astringent, cleansing, and skin regenerative. It is said to help prevent hair loss and thinning; it strengthens the hair. It also conditions hair, scalp, and skin, having a stimulating effect, especially when mixed with sage. Whether your skin is dry or oily, rosemary is good for inflamed scalp conditions such as dandruff or dermatitis.

Contraindications: Rosemary may be too stimulating for use during pregnancy. Those who have high blood pressure should also use rosemary with caution: It can raise the blood pressure.

SAGE

Sage oil is warming, spicy, herbaceous, and camphorlike. The oil is astringent, antiseptic, cleansing, and invigorating, stimulating blood circulation. It is effective in hair loss preparations and for sensitive skin conditions.

Contraindications: Sage should not be used by pregnant women or those who suffer from high blood pressure or epilepsy.

SANDALWOOD

The sweet, woody, exotic nature of this oil makes it very desirable for its fragrance alone. It is also moisturizing, skin regenerative, astringent, antiseptic, anti-inflammatory, and very soothing. It is well suited to all skin types — normal, oily, dry, mature. It has dynamic shine-enhancing properties for the hair.

TEA TREE

Clean, strong, and spicy, the aroma is slightly medicinal. Antiseptic and antifungal, the oil is effective for dandruff and for itchy or inflamed scalp

THYME

This oil is intense, with a sweet, spicy, herbaceous odor. Thyme is one of the most potent antiseptic oils available — so use it in moderation. It also stimulates blood circulation, invigorating the scalp, making this a desirable oil in hair loss or thinning formulas.

Contraindications: Not recommended for those who have high blood pressure.

YLANG-YLANG

This oil is sweet, floral, and very powerful. It is antiseptic, emollient, and quite moisture balancing. It normalizes sebum production and is thus well suited to all skin types — normal, oily, dry, and mature. It also stimulates the scalp, making it excellent for hair growth.

Contraindications: Ylang-ylang may be overly sedating for those with low blood pressure.

ORGANIC FOODSTUFFS

Many everyday ingredients can be used to create or enhance your hair care formulas — including some you probably never thought of! When you use any of the following, remember that what you ingest or apply topically to your body *becomes* your body. It's been proven that the skin has a high level of permeability; when you apply anything to your scalp, the possibility exists for some of that ingredient to be absorbed into your skin and bloodstream. Use only organic ingredients and you'll be sure that you are applying only the most healthful ingredients for your body.

APPLE CIDER VINEGAR

Vinegar is used to rinse the hair after shampooing, leaving it soft and shining. It will restore an acidic pH to the hair and skin, remove excess oil, remove soap residue, and help control dandruff flaking. Apple cider vinegar may be used on its own, or beneficial herbs may be steeped in it to add even more benefits to your rinse.

APPLE JUICE

Apples contain malic acid — a naturally occurring fruit acid. Used in small quantities, malic acid is moisturizing; in higher quantities, it is exfoliating.

AVOCADO

The flesh of this fruit is 75 percent unsaturated fat and up to 25 percent oil. Avocado is high in vitamins A, B, and C, as well as minerals, and is an excellent emollient and moisturizer for the hair and skin, particularly dry conditions.

BANANA

This fruit is high in carbohydrates; vitamins A, B, and C; and minerals, especially potassium. It has excellent humectant and moisturizing qualities for the hair.

BEER

The sugar and proteins in beer are tremendous for bodifying, or volumizing, the hair, adding manageability. It may be added to your shampoo or used as a final rinse.

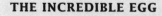

THE INCREDIBLE EGG

A raw egg (or two, depending on your hair length) left to dry in the hair and then shampooed out gives tremendous conditioning. This serves as a wonderful protein treatment to restore softness and manageability to your hair. You can do this once a month. I recommend that you use a final lemon juice or apple cider vinegar rinse to cut the film the egg leaves. (See page 114 and 116 for the details).

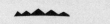

EGGS

These have a very high lecithin content, and lecithin has conditioning and moisturizing properties. Eggs are a hair strengthener, volumizer, and thickener. They are also a good emulsifier, binding ingredients together.

GELATIN

Gelatin will strengthen and fortify the hair because of its film-forming and thickening properties. Gelatin is purified protein derived from animal sources. If you prefer a vegetarian alternative, use pectin.

HONEY

High in vitamins and minerals, honey is made by bees from the nectar of flowering plants and trees. A very nutritive food when ingested, honey also has wonderful benefits for the skin and hair. Honey is a humectant and emollient, serving as a good moisturizer and conditioner.

MAYONNAISE

Whether you use an organic mayonnaise from the health food store or make your own, this mixture of egg yolk, vegetable oil, and lemon or vinegar has an emollient and smoothing effect on the hair. It's most effective when used as a hair pack or mask.

MILK

Milk is a rich source of protein, and contains high levels of vitamins A and D. Milk has tremendous emollient and moisturizing properties for the hair and skin.

SALT

High in minerals, salt has a softening and smoothing effect. It is astringent and antiseptic. It also accentuates the cleansing action of shampoos.

VODKA

Vodka is effective in removing buildup from the hair. It has astringent as well as oil-removing properties, making it effective in shampoos for oily hair or scalp.

WATER

This is one of the most often-used ingredients in hair and skin care products. In making your own formulas, use only distilled or purified water.

MIXING AND MATCHING

You may choose to add ingredients to the store-bought shampoos and conditioners that you are using. The ideal, of course, is to purchase the purest shampoos and conditioners that money can buy, then add desirable ingredients to them. Creating mixtures in a micro fashion (small batches) allows you to dabble from day to day or as your mood dictates. The following are some of my favorite formulas:

Egg. Mix 1 egg with ½ ounce (15 ml) of shampoo, or use a beaten egg by itself (2 if your hair is long). Massage this throughout your wet hair and the scalp, leave it on for a few minutes, and then rinse thoroughly with warm water.

Honey. A teaspoon (5 ml) of honey may be added to a teaspoon of shampoo, or use honey by itself as a wonderful hair pack and conditioner. Work ½ cup (120 ml; adjust the amount according to your hair length) through your hair lengths. Put a plastic shower cap or bag over the hair for 20 to 30 minutes to let your body heat optimize the conditioning benefit of the honey, then shampoo and rinse thoroughly.

Aloe vera. This incredibly healing and moisturizing plant substance has a normalizing effect for dry and oily conditions alike. Add a teaspoon (5 ml) of aloe to a teaspoon of shampoo and massage the shampoo in for a couple of minutes. Rinse thoroughly.

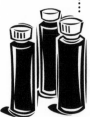

Plant oils. For dry hair or scalp conditions, add a teaspoon (5 ml) of any of the plant oils to a teaspoon of your regular shampoo.

Essential oils. Add up to a few drops to a tablespoon (15 ml) of shampoo, or 5 to 10 drops to an ounce (30 ml).

Gelatin. For a dynamic shot of fortifying protein, mix a pinch of gelatin into one application of shampoo; add 1 tablespoon (15 ml) to 8 ounces (235 ml) of shampoo; or mix a ¼-ounce (7 g) packet into a quart (1 liter) of water to use as a protein rinse.

CHAPTER 6

Making Your Own Shampoos and Conditioners

▼▼▼▼▼

This chapter will give you a road map to follow as you begin creating a wide range of hair care products and adapting them for your entire family. Remember that you can apply some of the principles and ideas discussed here to store-bought shampoos and conditioners. Also, some of the formulas you make yourself may nicely complement commercial products, and some of the ingredients I suggest for certain conditions may make wonderful additions to commercial products. Ultimately the way in which you integrate this information into your hair care routine is your own decision.

CHOOSING THE RIGHT INGREDIENTS

When making your own hair care formulas (or purchasing them from the store), you want to be sure that the ingredients you choose to use are the right ones for your particular hair condition. Many recipes call for a generic oil. That means that it's up to you to decide what your hair needs. Some guidelines are listed below, but be sure to review chapter 5 to understand the variables, and remember to look for natural, organic oils.

BASE OILS

Condition	Beneficial Oils
Normal scalp	Sunflower, almond, coconut, castor, or olive oil
Dry or sensitive scalp	Sunflower, almond, coconut, castor, or olive oil
Dry, brittle hair (including overstyled, permed, or color-treated)	Jojoba, sesame, or almond oil
Oily scalp and hair	Canola, safflower, sesame, or almond oil

Note: Those who suffer from dandruff will, depending on their condition, benefit from formulas designed for either dry scalps or oily scalps.

HERBS AND ESSENTIAL OILS

Condition	Beneficial Herbs	Beneficial Essential Oils
Normal hair and scalp	Calendula, chamomile, horsetail, nettle, rosemary, sage	Bergamot, carrot seed, cedarwood, chamomile, clary sage, cypress, geranium, juniper, lavender, lemon, neroli, orange, parsley seed, rose, rosemary, sage, sandalwood, thyme, ylang-ylang
Dry hair and scalp	Aloe, bay leaf, calendula, chamomile, coltsfoot, horsetail, lavender, marsh mallow, nettle	Carrot seed, cedarwood, chamomile, clary sage, geranium, jasmine, lavender, neroli, orange, parsley seed, rose, rosemary, sandalwood, ylang-ylang
Oily hair and scalp	Bay leaf, burdock, calendula, chamomile, horsetail, lemongrass, mint, nettle, thyme	Basil, bergamot, burdock, calendula, cedarwood, chamomile, cypress, eucalyptus, geranium, juniper, lavender, lemongrass, orange, peppermint, rose, rosemary, sage, thyme, ylang-ylang
Sensitive scalp (dandruff, dermatitis, inflammation)	Aloe, bay leaf, burdock, calendula, chamomile, horsetail, marsh mallow, nettle, oregano	Cedarwood, chamomile, clary sage, cypress, eucalyptus, jasmine, juniper, lavender, lemon, marjoram, neroli, orange, peppermint, rose, rosemary, sage, tea tree, thyme
Hair loss or thinning	Aloe, basil, bhringaraj, burdock, nettle, parsley, rosemary, sage	Bay, carrot seed, cedarwood, chamomile, clary sage, cypress, lavender, lemon, rosemary, sage, thyme, ylang-ylang
Blond hair (enhancing)	Calendula, chamomile, lemon	
Dark hair (enhancing)	Rosemary, sage, black tea	
Red hair (enhancing)	Henna, saffron (copper tones), sandalwood (reddish brown)	

Many recipes may also call for an unspecified essential oil, and in other cases you may decide to add a few drops of essential oil to a homemade or store-bought product. A few recipes even call for the herb of your choice. Your decision will be based upon the desired effect, whether physiological or psychological, from calming to stimulating or from balancing to moisturizing.

Use the lists on pages 103 and 104 as a way to assess the labels of products you purchase at health food, department, and drugstores as well as hair salons for the most healthful ingredients possible. Note that many herbs and essential oils cross over into different categories, showing the incredible diversity and efficacious nature of botanicals in beauty care.

OIL TREATMENTS FOR THE HAIR AND SCALP

Used for their stimulating, strengthening, and moisturizing properties, preshampoo scalp treatments loosen and slough off the dead surface cells on the scalp and provide nourishing emollient and antioxidant benefits. Oil treatments render the scalp more flexible, normalize both oily and dry itchy scalp conditions, and increase blood circulation to all the hair "roots." The protein and essential fatty acids found within these treatments will serve to fortify and smooth the hair while imparting a healthy shine. If you tend to use a lot of styling products, preshampoo oil treatments may have a softening effect on any film or buildup on your hair and scalp. These treatments are also especially beneficial for treating dandruff and dermatitis.

In contrast to most conditioners, which are applied after shampooing, hair and scalp oil treatments are generally administered before your bath or shower, when your hair is dry, and then shampooed from the hair. They can also be applied in the evening, left in overnight, and shampooed out the next morning, giving the oil a chance to provide optimal benefits. You will find that when you use an oil massage on a regular basis (which you should *not* do if you have oily hair and scalp or fine hair), your hair will not need an after-shampoo conditioner, but rather an after-shampoo hair rinse.

HAIR AND SCALP BOTANIC OIL TREATMENT

This soothing and simple treatment requires about 45 minutes of your time — most of it spent relaxing!

2 tablespoons (30 ml) vegetable, fruit, nut, herbal (page 107), or Ayurvedic (page 108) oil of your choice

15–30 drops essential oil of your choice (optional)

Yield: Enough for 1 application (if your hair is exceptionally thick or long, you may want to double the amounts)

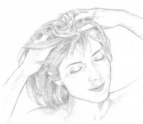
step 1

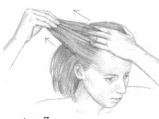
step 3

To make:

Thoroughly mix the oils in a plastic bottle with a flip-up spout top, or in a cup. Although you can certainly use it unheated, you may want to warm the oil by setting the container in hot water for a couple of minutes before using. Warming the oil will enhance your hair's ability to absorb it to a degree (although the true absorption of the oil is really related to its molecular makeup coupled with the degree of porosity of your hair).

To use:

1. Put some oil on your fingertips and work between your hands. Beginning at the top front hairline area, massage the oil with small circular strokes onto your scalp, working back toward the crown. Put more oil on your fingertips as needed.

2. Repeat this procedure from the temple area back to the lower crown, and through the nape area. Be gentle yet thorough, massaging your entire scalp for at least three minutes. Remember to massage with the pads of your fingertips in small circular movements along the scalp, not on top of the hair.

3. Next, put oil into your palms and work it between your hands. Massage this oil into the hair lengths from your scalp out to the ends with a gentle stroking or massaging motion.

4. Cover your hair with a plastic cap and close off with a clip. (Use and recycle a plastic bag from your whole food market, or try a reusable shower cap.) You can wrap a hot, damp towel around the plastic cap if you want to maximize the effect in the shortest amount of time (20 to

30 minutes). Or if time permits, take a bath, give yourself a face mask, meditate, or simply luxuriate around the house while your own body heat enhances the absorption of the treatment. Leaving the oil on for a longer period of time, even overnight, is also a possibility (pin up your oiled hair and sleep with a towel over your pillow).

5. Shampoo, condition with a detangling formula (especially useful for long hair) or herbal rinse if required, and then style.

6. If any of this recipe is left over, use it on your body. I like to work any extra oil into my elbows, or into my feet before covering them with organic cotton socks. If you opt to save the oil for another day, keep it refrigerated and use within three weeks.

HERBAL OIL

Herbalized or infused oils are chock full of all the goodness from both plant oils and specific herbs. These are potent! They're very effective for hair and scalp treatments. One of my favorite combinations for an herbalized oil is chamomile, rosemary, and horsetail with almond or sesame oil — this is a terrific conditioning oil for all hair and scalp types.

2–4 tablespoons (30–60 ml) dried herbs of your choice

1 cup (250 ml) base oil of your choice

Yield: Approximately 1 cup

To make:

1. Combine the ingredients in an airtight container. Let stand for several days (or even weeks, if time allows), stirring or gently shaking the mixture frequently.

2. Strain off the oil and discard the spent herbs. Store in dark glass bottles in a cool, dark place. Will keep for 3 to 4 weeks.

To use:

Use as an oil treatment for your hair and massage (as described on page 106), or as a massage oil for your body.

AYURVEDIC OIL

This is a traditional Ayurvedic approach to making and using oils. Use the herb bhringaraj, called "ruler of the hair" in Ayurveda, to create a highly effective medicated oil that is famous in India for removing grayness and reversing hair loss, or select your favorite herb(s) and use in combination with Bhringaraj or other herbs to create your own uniquely individualized herbal oil.

¼ cup (60 ml) dried herbs of your choice
1 cup (250 ml) water
2 cups (500 ml) sesame oil
3–5 drops essential oils of your choice (optional)

Yield: Approximately 2 cups (500 ml)

To make:

1. Combine the herbs and water in a stainless-steel or glass pan. Bring to a boil, reduce the heat, and then simmer, uncovered, until approximately half of the liquid has evaporated. Strain the herbs off.

2. Add the decoction to the sesame oil in a stainless-steel pan, bring to a boil, then immediately turn the flame down as low as possible and let this mixture simmer very slowly for at least an hour. The oil will be ready when all of the liquid from the decoction has evaporated and a drop of water dropped into the oil makes a crackling sound.

3. You can add a few drops of essential oils as desired. Store this oil in an airtight amber bottle.

To use:

Use for scalp and hair massages as described on pages 106–107.

SHAMPOO FORMULAS

While conditioners are of primary importance for the hair, shampoos are of primary importance for the scalp. Of course, when giving yourself a shampoo, you work the lather through the lengths of hair, which will help remove styling products if you tend to use a lot of them. However, your goal should be to massage and cleanse the scalp, removing dead skin cells, sweat, pollution, and excess oil while encouraging the flow of nutrient rich blood to the hair roots.

There are two different approaches to creating your own personalized shampoos. One is to add nutritive ingredients to a pure shampoo or castile or liquid glycerin soap that you purchase. The other method is to entirely create your own. Whichever you decide upon, choose the herbs or essential oils according to your scalp and hair type (see page 104).

(see page 104)

> ### SOAP DEFINITIONS
>
> A **castile** soap is a mild soap made from olive oil. A **glycerin** soap is an effective moisturizing base to which you can add your herbal preparation or essential oils.

SOAPWORT SHAMPOO

This is an excellent all-purpose shampoo for all types of scalp and hair. It does not have tremendous lather, but it cleanses very well and has no chemicals whatsoever. Many Native American tribes used the root of soapwort to wash their hair. You may choose to infuse a couple of tablespoons (30 ml) of your favorite herbs along with the soapwort, if desired.

1 ounce (30 g) soapwort root

12 ounces (354 ml) of purified water

1 teaspoon (5 ml) base oil of your choice

15–60 drops essential oils of your choice, as conditions require

Yield: 10–12 ounces (295–354 ml)

To make:
1. Crush the soapwort root in a mortar and pestle (or with the flat side of a wooden spoon or large knife).
2. Place the crushed root in the water in a stainless-steel pan. Bring to a boil, reduce the heat, and simmer for approximately 10 minutes. Remove from the heat, cool, then strain the liquid into an airtight bottle with a nozzle on top for dispensing.
3. Add the base and essential oils to the container. Shake well before each use. This shampoo will keep for up to a week if refrigerated.

To use:
Shampoo, then follow with an herbal vinegar rinse.

Oily scalp: You can eliminate the base oil from this shampoo if your scalp tends to be very oily.

PURE SHAMPOO

The ingredients for this recipe are chosen for their desirable aromatic as well as therapeutic values. Some of my favorite formulations for specific conditions are outlined below. I encourage you to experiment with the herbs, essential oils, and other ingredients I've discussed so far, though, because the possible variations are tremendous.

1–2 tablespoons (15–30 ml) dried herbs of your choice (see suggestions on page 111)

8 ounces (235 ml) purified water

2 ounces (60 ml) liquid castile or glycerin soap

1 teaspoon (5 ml) base oil of your choice (eliminate or reduce for oily conditions; increase for dry; see chart on page 111

15–60 drops essential oils of your choice, as conditions require

Yield: 8–10 ounces (235–295 ml)

To make:

1. Create a decoction or infusion of your desired herb or combinations of herbs. Remember that a decoction is used for roots, stems, and seeds, or more fibrous, tough plants, while infusions are used for more delicate plant parts, including leaves and flowers. If you are combining herbs that need different treatments, decoct and infuse them separately, then mix the herbalized liquids.

For a decoction, place the herbs in water in a stainless-steel or glass pan. Bring to a boil, reduce the heat, and simmer on low for up to 10 minutes. Remove from the heat, let the mixture cool, strain off the liquid, and discard the spent herbs.

For an infusion, bring the water to a boil. Place the herbs in a stainless-steel or glass pan and pour the boiling water over them. Let steep for at least 20 minutes, then let the mixture cool (if it isn't cool already), strain off the liquid, and discard the spent herbs.

Tip: To increase the potency of the formula, let the herbs steep in the cooled liquid in an airtight container for a couple of days before straining and using.

2. Mix the herbal infusion or decoction with the soap, base oil, and desired essential oils. Shake well. Refrigerate the shampoo between uses, for up to a week, then discard. Adding 1 teaspoon (5 ml) of vodka to this mixture will add 2 to 3 weeks to its shelf life, as will adding

1 teaspoon (5 ml) of either vitamin E or wheat germ oil.

To use:

Use the formula for every shampoo (see the eight-step instructions on pages 80–82). Shake well before each use.

Additives: You can also add ingredients with properties (as described in chapter 5) suitable for your particular hair condition, such as apple juice, honey, egg, aloe vera, gelatin, glycerin, or lecithin. Use 1 tablespoon (15 ml) per shampoo formula.

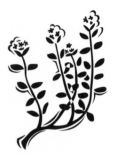

PURE SHAMPOO FOR DIFFERENT CONDITIONS

Note: This gives you a framework from which to make your own formulas. It is not necessary to use every ingredient I've outlined. If you choose to decoct only one specific herb for a given condition, and add one favored essential oil, that's perfectly all right. The fact that you are using a pure shampoo with no chemicals in it is the first step toward becoming as creative as you would like. Also remember that you can do something as simple as purchasing a pure shampoo and add healthful ingredients as required — such as essential oils, egg, or gelatin. Remember to complete a patch test before using your hair care formula (see page 93).

Condition	Herbs to Decoct or Infuse	Base Oils	Essential Oils
Normal hair	Horsetail, nettle, rosemary	Almond oil plus up to 1 tablespoon (15 ml) of aloe vera	Bergamot, orange, rose
Dry hair	Horsetail, lavender, watercress	Jojoba oil plus up to 1 tablespoon (15 ml) of aloe vera and lecithin (drizzle into warmed formula)	Carrot seed, clary sage, geranium, jasmine
Oily hair	Burdock, lemongrass, thyme	Almond oil	Basil, peppermint, rosemary
Sensitive scalp (dandruff, dermatitis, inflammation)	Burdock, chamomile, horsetail	Jojoba or castor oil	Cedarwood, rosemary, sage, tea tree
Hair loss or thinning	Basil, rosemary, sage	Jojoba oil	Cedarwood, clary sage, ylang-ylang

HAIR RINSES

Herbal hair rinses are by nature conditioning and serve a variety of functions. When applied through your hair after shampooing they will close down the cuticle, creating exceptionally smooth and shiny hair that feels thicker and is more manageable. Hair rinses can also be quite therapeutic for the scalp. Depending on the ingredients you choose, they can also detangle the hair, return it to an acid-balanced pH, remove soap residue, and enhance color.

A hair rinse may be as simple as adding a few drops of an essential oil to your final rinse water for its aromatic and therapeutic value, or as complex as creating a medicinal rinse that combines several herbs and essential oils. Many options exist. The type of rinse that you choose to make will depend on how creative you want to get. Your choice of herbs and essential oils will depend on your condition or problem. Again, you will want to refer to the ingredients listings in chapter 5 to select the herbs, essential oils, and natural ingredients that resonate with your needs and desires.

WHEN SHOULD I RINSE?

- If you have normal to dry hair, use the rinse before applying a conditioner.
- If you have oily hair, use the rinse after applying a conditioner.

Application of Rinses

Hair rinses can be left in the hair or rinsed out, depending on the nature of your condition. For example, rinses for scalp conditions like dandruff and dermatitis are best left in the hair and looked upon as treatments that are used several times to normalize or balance the condition. On the other hand, vinegar rinses are generally washed from the hair. Your reasons for using a hair rinse will determine the best place for application and how long you should leave it on.

If you're going to rinse the application from your hair, blot your hair dry with a towel, then apply the rinse from a spout bottle. Distribute evenly through your hair, massage through the hair lengths, and leave on for approximately 5 minutes before rinsing with cool to tepid water.

If you're leaving the rinse in your hair, first gently towel-blot your hair, then wrap a towel around your neck. Leaning over a sink or basin, apply the rinse with a spout bottle. For extra potency, pour over a basin so the rinse won't drain away, then pour the collected liquid through the hair to use every drop of the rinse. Blot dry with a towel and proceed with styling.

Rinse Recipes

Now that you have dabbled in creating customized shampoos, let's look at using herbal rinses for a variety of treatments.

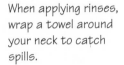

When applying rinses, wrap a towel around your neck to catch spills.

HERBAL INFUSION RINSE

You can use the suggested herbs singly or in combination.

2 tablespoons (30 ml) dried herbs (see suggestions below)
1 cup (250 ml) purified water
3–5 drops essential oils of your choice (optional)

Yield: 1 treatment

To make:
1. Bring the water to a boil. Place the herbs in a stainless-steel or glass pan and pour the boiling water over them. Let steep for 10–15 minutes.
2. Drain off the liquid and discard the spent herbs. Mix in the essential oil and then use immediately.
To use:
Apply as directed on page 112–113.

Herbs for normal hair and scalp: Chamomile, horsetail, rosemary, and sage.
Herbs for oily hair and scalp: Horsetail, lemongrass, mint, and thyme.
Herbs for dry hair and scalp: Horsetail, lavender, marsh mallow, and watercress.

SENSITIVE, ITCHY SCALP RINSE

The following herbal combination is antiseptic, astringent, and soothing. Tea tree essential oil is antifungal and antibacterial and so very effective for scalp problems that have a fungal or bacterial origin.

2 cups (500 ml) purified or distilled water

1 heaping tablespoon (15 ml, or about 1 handful) each of dried nettles, rosemary, and sage

1 drop tea tree essential oil (optional)

1 drop lavender essential oil

Yield: 1–3 treatments, depending on hair length

To make:
Place the herbs in the water in a stainless-steel or glass pan. Bring to a boil, then immediately remove from the heat. Let the "tea" sit overnight, then strain out the herbs.

To use:
After shampooing with a gentle shampoo and rinsing thoroughly, apply the herbal tea as your final rinse as instructed on page 112–113.

RINSE TIP

I like to keep rinses in color application bottles. These have a narrow spout on the end for a controlled, even distribution of the rinse through the hair. You can purchase them at beauty supply stores.

LEMON JUICE HIGHLIGHTING RINSE

This rinse makes the hair very shiny, and is great for bringing out highlights in blond hair — although it's wonderful for all hair colors. It is most beneficial for normal to oily hair conditions.

2 lemons

2 cups (500 ml) purified water

Yield: 1 treatment

To make and use:
Squeeze the juice from the lemons into the water. Work through the hair as instructed on page 112–113. Rinse, if desired. Left in hair, the formula accentuates the acidification of both hair and scalp, softening and subtly lightening the hair.

NETTLES BODIFYING HAIR RINSE

A nettles hair rinse is great as a bodifying treatment and will add strength, luster, and incredible fullness to overworked hair. Adjust the amount of water and nettles according to the length of your hair. A few drops of lavender essential oil will provide not only fragrance, but also shine and silkiness to your hair.

2–4 tablespoons (30–60 ml) dried nettles

1 cup (250 ml) purified or distilled water

3–5 drops lavender essential oil (optional)

Yield: 1 treatment

To make:
Combine the herbs and water in a stainless-steel or glass pan. Bring to a boil, reduce the heat, and simmer, covered, for half an hour. Remove from the heat and let cool, then strain out the liquid and discard the spent herbs.

To use:
Use after shampooing as instructed on pages 112–113. Do not rinse out.

Tincture tip: You can also make this recipe with a tincture of nettles. Add approximately 30 drops to 1 cup (235 ml) of water and apply as a rinse.

FORTIFYING PROTEIN RINSE

This formula fortifies the hair and smoothes its cuticle layer.

1¼-ounce (7 g) package gelatin

2 cups (500 ml) water

Yield: 1–3 treatments, depending on hair length

To make and use:
Mix the gelatin into the water. Work through your hair as described on pages 112–113, until your hair is totally saturated. Leave on for 10 to 15 minutes, then rinse.

RESTORATIVE APPLE CIDER VINEGAR RINSE

▼▼▼

This rinse closes the cuticle layer, creating great shine, softness, and manageability. Organic apple cider vinegar has astringent and toning properties. It has a very normalizing effect and will restore the hair's natural acid mantle. It's especially good for oily scalp and hair conditions.

2 tablespoons
(30 ml) apple
cider vinegar
1 cup (250 ml)
purified water
3–5 drops essential
oils of your choice
(optional)

Yield: 1 treatment

To make:
Combine all ingredients.
To use:
After every shampoo, apply the rinse as instructed on pages 112–113. Rinse with cool to tepid water (you may want to leave it in for oilier hair or scalp types).

APPLE CIDER DANDRUFF TREATMENT

▼▼▼

Apples contain malic acid, an alpha hydroxy acid, which works as an exfoliant and emollient to lift dandruff away from the scalp. This treatment will not only control flaking scalp but moisturize as well. Apply after shampooing and conditioning.

½ cup (125 ml) apple
cider (preferably
organic)

To use:
Massage the cider into the scalp area with your fingertips. Repeat after every shampoo; you will see significant results after a week's time. Repeat treatment whenever outbreaks of dandruff occur.

HERBAL VINEGAR RINSE FOR SENSITIVE SCALP

This medicinal vinegar is great to have on hand for an itchy, sensitive scalp, or for dandruff problems. It may even prevent dandruff because of the balancing effect that acidic vinegar has on the scalp. Antimicrobial herbs such as oregano and lavender will make for a more powerful and pleasant-smelling remedy. Note that oregano is a great detangler for the hair, as is rosemary. Naturally, you could choose a variety of different herbs, depending on the effect that you are looking for.

¼ cup (60 ml) fresh oregano

¼ cup (60 ml) fresh lavender buds (or 2 tablespoons — 30 ml — dried)

2 cups (500 ml) organic apple cider vinegar

Yield: Approximately 15 treatments

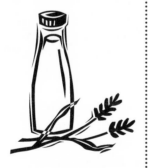

To make:

1. Chop the oregano and the lavender buds. Place them in a widemouthed quart (1 liter) glass jar and pour in the apple cider vinegar, making sure that the herbs are completely covered (add more vinegar if necessary). Gently stir, then cover. If you're using a metal lid, place plastic wrap or wax paper over the opening first, then cover, so that the vinegar doesn't corrode the metal.

2. Let the herbs steep in the vinegar for up to two weeks at room temperature. Then strain off the liquid, discard the spent herbs, and store the vinegar in a dark glass bottle in a cool, dark place. This herbal remedy will keep for up to a year.

To use:

Add 2 tablespoons (30 ml) of the herbal vinegar to 1 cup (250 ml) of warm water and massage into your scalp after shampooing. Do not rinse out. You may do this once a week, or more if required.

PURIFYING AND STIMULATING HAIR AND SCALP RINSE

This herbal vinegar rinse has a soothing and detoxifying effect on the hair and scalp while it increases the blood circulation to the hair follicles.

2 tablespoons (30 ml) dried mint
2 tablespoons (30 ml) dried basil
2 tablespoons (30 ml) dried rosemary
2 tablespoons (30 ml) dried sage
3-5 drops essential oils of your choice (try a few drops each of lavender and peppermint)
2 cups (500 ml) organic apple cider vinegar

Yield: Approximately 15 treatments

To make:

1. Chop the herbs. Place them in a wide-mouthed quart (1 liter) glass jar and pour in the apple cider vinegar, making sure that the herbs are completely covered (add more vinegar if necessary). Gently stir, then cover. If you're using a metal lid, place plastic wrap or wax paper over the opening first, then cover, so that the vinegar doesn't corrode the metal.

2. Let the herbs steep in the vinegar for up to two weeks at room temperature. Then strain off the liquid, discard the spent herbs, and store the vinegar in a dark glass bottle in a cool, dark place. This remedy will keep for up to a year.

To use:

Add 2 tablespoons (30 ml) of the herbal vinegar to 1 cup (250 ml) of warm water and massage into your scalp after shampooing. Do not rinse out. Repeat once every week.

For hair loss or thinning: Apply treatment every day for 1 week, and once a week thereafter.

HAIR COLOR RINSES

Use the following herbal decoctions as color-enhancing rinses after shampooing and rinsing. Towel-dry your hair, then flow the rinse through it. Do not rinse out. (I will revisit this subject in chapter 9 when I discuss color — along with more natural coloring options.)

◆ For enhancing blond hair, decoct calendula and chamomile.
◆ For enhancing dark hair, decoct rosemary, sage, or black tea.
◆ For enhancing red hair, decoct sandalwood (for reddish brown tones) or saffron (for copper tones).

BODIFYING BEER HAIR RINSE

My mother turned me on to this when I was a teenager, and it really does work. It must be the hops, barley, and malt — all that sugar and protein. It gives hair incredible body and fullness.

1 12-ounce (355 ml) bottle or can of beer

Yield: 1–2 treatments, depending on hair length

To make and use:
Pour the beer into a glass or container and let sit until it is flat and at room temperature. After shampooing and rinsing, work the beer through your hair (as described on pages 112–113). Do not rinse out; the beer smell will dissipate as your hair dries and you'll be left with lush, bouncy hair.

Note: If your tastes lean more toward champagne, you can use champagne for the same type of bodifying result.

HAIR AND SCALP CONDITIONERS

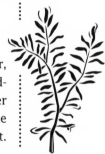

Conditioning treatments strengthen and moisturize the hair, complementing the acidifying nature of hair rinses. Depending on the treatment, they can be applied before or after shampooing and can be rinsed out or left in. Generally, the longer conditioners are left in, the more powerful their effect.

ALL-PURPOSE CONDITIONER

This conditioner is especially good for maintaining healthy, normal hair in its optimal condition. Aloe vera has tremendous moisturizing properties, while lemon juice is quite purifying and cleansing. I suggest using lavender, rosemary, or mint essential oils, depending upon whether you're seeking a relaxing or stimulating effect.

¼ cup (60 ml) aloe vera gel
½ lemon
3–5 drops essential oils of your choice

Yield: 1 treatment

To make:
Mix the aloe vera gel with the juice of half a lemon. Add the essential oils.

To use:
Apply to freshly shampooed hair. Leave on for 3 to 5 minutes, then rinse thoroughly.

STIMULATING GINGER ELIXIR SCALP TREATMENT

Ginger is considered one of the most powerful herbs in Ayurveda. It has potent stimulating properties, increasing the blood circulation. This is an excellent moisturizing scalp conditioning formula which can stimulate hair growth.

1 tablespoon (15 ml) finely grated ginger

1 tablespoon (15 ml) sesame or jojoba oil

Yield: 1 treatment

To make and use:
This formula can be applied either before or after shampooing. If applied after, be sure to rinse extremely well. Combine the ingredients, massage into the scalp, and leave on for at least 30 minutes. (You can leave on overnight to receive the maximum benefit.) Rinse out with tepid water.

DEEP PROTEIN CONDITIONING TREATMENT

Gelatin is essentially animal protein. In this treatment, gelatin is used to fortify and strengthen the hair. This treatment is especially good for dry, fragile, or brittle hair types.

1 tablespoon (15 ml) gelatin

1 cup (250 ml) purified water

1 teaspoon (5 ml) organic apple cider vinegar

2 drops each jasmine, clary sage, and rosemary essential oils

Yield: 1 treatment

To make and use:
Mix the gelatin with the water, and let it slightly gel (do not let it set all the way). Add the apple cider vinegar and the essential oils and mix well. Work through freshly shampooed hair, leave on for 5 to 10 minutes, and rinse thoroughly. You can repeat this treatment once a week.

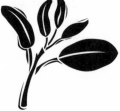

Soothing Leave-In Conditioner for All Hair Types

This leave-in conditioner imparts wonderful shine and makes the hair silky, smooth, and manageable. The fragrance is calming and soothing.

2 cups (500 ml) purified or distilled water
1 tablespoon (15 ml) dried comfrey
½ tablespoon (8 ml) dried chamomile
½ tablespoon (8 ml) dried calendula
15–20 drops essential oils of your choice (optional)

Yield: 8–12 treatments, depending on hair length

To make:

1. Bring the water to a boil. Place the herbs in a stainless-steel or glass pan and pour the boiling water over them. Let steep until cooled.

2. Strain the liquid into a clean spray bottle and discard the spent herbs. Mix in the essential oils. My favorite combination for this formula is 5 drops each of neroli, lavender, sandalwood, and rosemary. Shake well. Keep this formula refrigerated between uses. Use this within a couple of weeks of making, then make a new batch.

To use:

Spray this onto your hair after shampooing and towel drying.

For extra conditioning: You can add a teaspoon (5 ml) of panthenol (vitamin B$_5$), a substantive and hair-strengthening vitamin available at most health food stores, to this formula for extra conditioning benefits.

Stimulating Leave-In Conditioner for All Hair Types

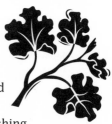

Follow the same directions as above, but instead of floral herbs substitute the aromatic oregano, basil, and rosemary. Also, add essential oils of bergamot, clary sage, and geranium. These herbs and oils have a refreshing, stimulating aroma.

MAYO HAIR DRESSING

This is one of the simplest yet most effective conditioners for the hair. It is especially effective for dry hair. You can use organic mayonnaise purchased from the whole food store, or make your own (my husband, James, shares his mayonnaise recipe with us below). Mayonnaise will feed the hair nutritious eggs, vegetable oil, vinegar, and lemon juice. Add a couple of drops each of sage, rosemary, and thyme essential oils to the mayo if desired before working it into your hair. Keep some mayo aside, of course, to make a deluxe deli sandwich within the next couple of days!

2 egg yolks

1 cup (235 ml) canola or olive oil

¼ teaspoon (1 ml) dry mustard

½ teaspoon (2.5 ml) sea salt

½ teaspoon (2.5 ml) apple cider vinegar or lemon juice

½ teaspoon (2.5 ml) confectioners' sugar

1½ tablespoons (23 ml) plus 1 teaspoon (5 ml) apple cider vinegar

2 tablespoons (30 ml) lemon juice

Yield: 1 treatment

1. Set out the egg yolks and oil until they are at room temperature.

2. With a whisk, beat the yolks until they reach a lemony color. Beat in the mustard, sea salt, ½ teaspoon (2.5 ml) apple cider vinegar, and confectioners' sugar. Slowly beat in half of the canola or olive oil. The mixture will begin to thicken and emulsify.

3. In a separate bowl, combine the apple cider vinegar with the lemon juice. Add this mixture alternatively with the remaining ½ cup (120 ml) of canola or olive oil into the mayonnaise mixture by whisking them in drop by drop. Mix until the ingredients have been totally beaten in to create a thick mayo mixture.

To use: Massage mayonnaise liberally through your hair. Place a plastic bag over your hair and leave it on for 15 to 30 minutes. Shampoo, rinse, and follow with a fragrant essential oil hair rinse.

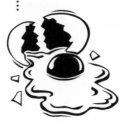

Avocado Dry Hair Conditioner

This treatment is exceptional for dry hair. Avocado has a high vitamin and mineral content, and tremendous emollience and moisturizing ability — especially when blended with the oils in this formula.

½ ripe avocado
1 teaspoon (5 ml) wheat germ oil
1 teaspoon (5 ml) jojoba oil

Yield: 1 treatment

To make and use:
Combine all ingredients. Work the mixture through your shampooed hair and scalp. Cover your hair with a plastic bag to allow for your body heat to accentuate the conditioning effect, and leave the mixture on for 15 to 30 minutes. Rinse thoroughly.

Moisturizing Banana Hair Conditioner

High in vitamins, and minerals, bananas are very effective humectants and moisturizers. Couple this with honey and sweet almond oil and you have a match made in heaven.

1 small, ripe organic banana
1 tablespoon (15 ml) organic honey
1 teaspoon (5 ml) sweet almond oil

Yield: 1 treatment

To make and use:
Mash the banana together with the honey and sweet almond oil. Apply this mixture to your shampooed hair. Cover your hair with a plastic bag to allow for body heat to accentuate the conditioning effect, and leave the mixture on for 15 to 30 minutes. Rinse thoroughly.

CHAPTER 7
Personalizing Your Cut and Style

▼▼▼▼

Depending on your hair type, texture, and condition, as well as what you desire as a "look," by working with your hairstylist you will be able to determine the hairstyle that is going to be the easiest for you to manage, and that captures your own personal sense of style. Now, this is no small undertaking. A naturally healthy hairstyle usually means a cut that does not require a lot of products to stay in place or to be manageable. Your haircut is the foundation of your hairstyle. If the haircut is personalized for you — your hair type, texture, and condition, and your lifestyle — then you should not have to use large amounts of products or styling tools to get your hair to look good.

Please don't misunderstand me. It's okay to use styling products and to blow-dry your hair. It's all a matter of degree. As in life, all things in moderation is how you keep your balance.

THE CUT CREATES THE STYLE

Hair reflects our individuality, and it is a deeply organic part of the body that can speak volumes about how we feel about ourselves. The shape or form of the style will be dependent on the haircut. When I cut clients' hair, I first speak to them at length about what their expectations are. Some of the questions I ask my clients, and questions you should ask yourself, are:

- Do you have any particular likes or dislikes about your hair?
- What are you willing to do at home to keep the style looking its best?
- How much time do you have to work with it?
- What are you willing to use, product-wise, to change the grain of the fabric, so to speak?

I also look at their anatomy — their height, weight, head shape, face shape — and note facial features in order to play up the most dynamic ones (for example, vibrant eyes, high cheekbones, or full lips), while camouflaging certain others (such as a high or low forehead, short neck, large nose or ears, or wide face).

Working with Your Natural Features

Illusion styling is the process of shifting the weight and length of hair based on your natural features to effect a desirable change. Counterbalance is the key to creating these desirable accents and effects. Here are some of the basics:

Balancing your features. The size and shape of your face should be complemented and balanced by the shape of your haircut.

Proportion. Petite bodies appear even smaller with large or excessively long hairstyles, and large bodies will look still larger with a hairstyle too short or close to the head. Depending on your body size and height, your hairstyle should be in balance with the rest of your body.

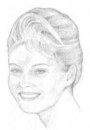

A wide face can be balanced accordingly with closeness on the sides and fullness on top.

Fringe. A fringe, or bangs, should be used to accentuate your eyes. Too long or too thick a fringe will de-emphasize the eyes and accentuate your nose, making your face look smaller. However, a fringe at the right length can bring out your eyes.

Part. A center part can be worn by very few people (except for young children or adolescents). A side part or no part is preferable; or add a soft fringe (bangs).

Length. Longer hair should be either below the shoulder blades or above the shoulders to create a free-moving clear line that has fullness. Shorter hair will expose more of the facial features and neck and shoulder structure

Styling direction. Graduated or layered hair that is brushed back off the face creates a fuller shape that can enhance the facial features. Layered hair that is styled forward onto the face is generally not practical for most people.

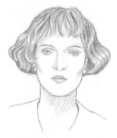

A long face can be balanced with diminished volume on top and width placed at sides.

Cut Considerations

When pondering what type of haircut you want to fulfill your expectations and needs, there are three major considerations:

- Line: The outer frame of the cut
- Shape: The dimensional form of the cut
- Length: from short to medium to long, and all lengths in-between

Above all, be sure to get a trim at least every 6 to 8 weeks. This will keep the line and shape of your style looking clean and fresh. More importantly, it will get rid of any split ends before they have a chance to split upward along the hair strand. Nothing gets rid of split ends except trimming them off. (Products that claim to get rid of them are simply "gluing" the split ends back together.)

THE LINE OF THE HAIRCUT

From the front hairline through the sides to the back, the outer or perimeter frame of the cut gives every hairstyle a distinctive look. Once you understand that there is a difference in how the various types of lines fall and move depending on the length, shape, and texture of your hair, you will be able to more readily ask for what you want in the perimeter frame of your cut.

Types of Lines

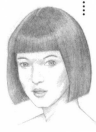

A horizontal line at the fringe and through the sides creates the classic bob cut.

The line that is cut may be blunt and exact, soft and wispy, or perhaps even textured and chunky. The effect or quality of this line will change depending on the texture of your hair, whether the line is cut close to or far away from your hairline, and direction in which the line travels — horizontally or diagonally, straight or curved.

Horizontal lines. A horizontal line has great stability, and doesn't really allow for much directional movement (a flow backward or forward) of the hair.

Diagonal lines. Diagonal lines can create a directional flow, forward or backward, in the hair. A diagonally backward line can be a desirable cut to have when you like to wear your hair back away from the face — depending on the type of shape that has been cut, you can also wear it in its natural fall or softly blown-dried forward for variety.

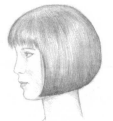

A slight diagonal forward line (left) creates a flowing-forward movement in the hair, while a diagonal back line (right) creates a flowing-backward movement.

Rounded lines. Rounded or curved lines around the front hairline area can be cut just at the fringe area, or they can curve around and into the side area, where they continue to flow back or perhaps blend with another line at the side area. They are also frequently used at the nape area.

Lines and Hairlines

The shorter the line is cut around the hairline area, the more the features are exposed. Keep this in mind, because it requires a certain level of self-confidence to wear a very short length around the perimeter hairline area — although I have to admit that very short hair all over can be quite freeing. One quick point on short hair, for men and women alike: Try to have the back neckline, when cut short, work as much with your natural neckline and growth patterns as possible. To razor or clipper the natural hairline unnecessarily high not only looks unnatural but requires diligent upkeep.

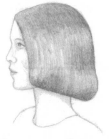

A concave rounded line at the fringe can blend into layers at the side.

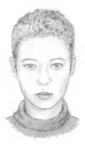

Very short hair requires very little maintenance.

THE SHAPE OF THE HAIRCUT

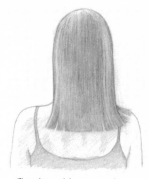

This long blunt cut has a horizontal weight line.

There are only four ways that the hair can be cut — and once you know these four haircuts, you'll understand that every possible haircut that can be created is simply a combination of them. They are *the blunt cut* (all one length), *the graduated cut* (angled or stacked out along the edges), *progressive layers* (layers that move from short to long), and *uniform layers* (layers that are even in their length). Very simply, blunt and graduated cuts lend solidity and weightiness. Layered shapes allow for more airiness, fullness, and volume.

The Blunt Cut

Also called the bob, this haircut is a modern classic! Blunt cuts can be done for all types of hair, whether short, medium, long, straight, wavy, or curly. All the lengths fall to the same line, called the weight line. The hair is held straight down by the natural fall of gravity and the cut. The blunt-cut line may be horizontal, diagonal backward or forward, or curved.

One of the biggest benefits of the blunt cut is that it provides an easy-care, easy-wear hairstyle. It's a great cut for fine, medium, or coarse hair; it's actually a preferred cut for fine, straight hair because it creates a sense of fullness and shiny sleekness. On curly hair, it is important to understand that when dry, an all one-length haircut will expand out into an exaggerated triangular shape. If you do not want this effect, then graduate the bottom edge of the line or place some long layers over it to soften and round off the strong angular weight corner.

Rounding off the corner of a blunt cut is a very modern way to soften the angular effect of a blunt cut on any type of hair texture — straight, wavy, or curly.

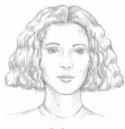

Before

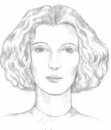

After

The Graduated Cut

The graduated cut is another popular style worn worldwide by women and men. In this technique, hair is cut away from the head at an angle so that it stacks up and out along an angled line. Remember Dorothy Hamill's wedge from the Olympic ice-skating arena? This is a very easy style to wear and care for. The graduation allows for movement and volume, depending on the length and the natural or introduced textural movement in the hair.

Graduation happens around the perimeter frame of the cut in horizontal, diagonal forward, or diagonal back lines. Graduation works best on hair that has some body to it, as some volume will accentuate the shape (in order to be low-maintenance wash and wear). Most people with medium or fine straight hair who want a graduated cut must be willing to use styling products to enhance movement and body.

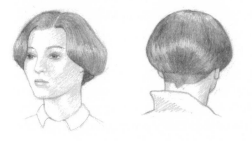

Graduation can be applied in various degrees. The cut on the left shows a low degree of graduation along a diagonal back line; the cut on the right shows a high degree of graduation at the neck line below an overhanging horizontal blunt cut.

VIDEO IMAGING YOUR NEXT HAIRSTYLE?

Blonde, brunette, redhead, straight, wavy, curly, long, medium, short — can you see yourself wearing styles that have any or all these qualities? Video imaging is wild and fantastic! A photo portrait is taken of you and fed into the system; then the hairstylist can place on the monitor a variety of styles that you've selected from a portfolio. The technology is so advanced and the effect so real that you can virtually see yourself with each style, then work with your hairstylist to determine which look is best for you.

Progressive Layers

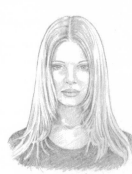

Progressive layers simply refers to layers that move from shorter to longer. This is a classic type of cutting technique that has been around for quite some time. Progressive layers are generally cut through the interior area of the hair and fall over a perimeter frame that has been cut blunt or graduated. This technique requires that your hairstylist knows exactly how you want the layers to fall, because so many variations are possible.

Progressive layers can be restricted to the front hairline area to frame the face.

Layering for volume. Given a certain amount of wave in the hair, layering the hair is the number one way to give it volume. Be aware that short progressive layers on very curly hair can create a bizarre big-head shape — I usually do not recommend layering very curly hair, unless it will be done with extreme subtlety. You can, of course, layer straight hair, but understand that in order to attain volume on this type of haircut you will need to blow-dry it with a vented or round brush, and possibly use a curling iron or hot rollers to achieve more fullness and textural movement.

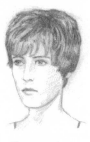

Progressive layers can create volume for straight hair.

Directional layering. Layers can also be cut to create directional movement, whether horizontal, diagonal forward, or diagonal back. Horizontal layers fall evenly and horizontally across the hair. These layers are shorter at the center top of the head and increase in length outward toward the perimeter frame area. They may be cut to mirror or flow along a perimeter frame line that has been cut horizontally, or cut without regard for the perimeter frame line.

Diagonal layers flow diagonally forward or backward, framing the face or falling back away from it.

The horizontal layers at left mimic the horizontal line at the bottom edge of the hair shape, while the short diagonal layers at right encourage the hair to fall back from the face.

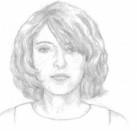 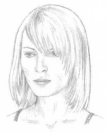

Layering around the face. Layering around the face has many variations and can be used to accentuate your natural features; it combines particularly well with blunt cuts. Slide cutting (see box) is a particularly effective technique for creating these layers.

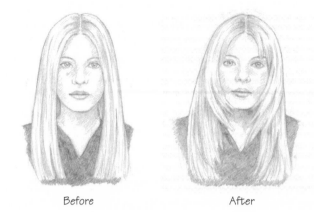

Before   After

One of my favorite methods for layering around the face is to bring all lengths forward and angle the line outward, from short to long, softly framing the face.

SLIDE CUTTING

A classic technique for progressive layering is slide cutting. Here, open shears are used to glide and cut along the desired line, creating very quick length increases. This is for those of you who perhaps have a very short fringe but very long perimeter lengths, and who want some form of blending between these two contrasting lengths or shapes. For layering around the face, such blending takes place only around the front hairline area. This technique may also be used through the interior area (again, by someone who is well qualified) to create a dramatic length increase from any shorter interior areas outward to the longer perimeter frame. This is not like conventional layering; it's a technique for those who want to keep the maximum amount of length and weight around the perimeter frame area, yet would like to have a certain amount of textural movement along the top surface. It is also the best way to connect areas that are cut very differently in their shape and length.

Uniform Layers

Uniform layers are used for both men's and women's cuts. All lengths are brought straight out from the curve of the head and cut evenly. It may be used throughout the entire cut or throughout the interior area of a cut to fall over a graduated cut around the perimeter frame.

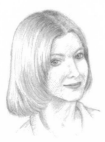

Short uniform layers work on straight and wavy hair alike. A small amount of styling lotion worked through straight hair can help in blow-drying this shape into place, or you can simply mold the hair into place and let it dry. Because of the roundness of this shape, it will be quite expansive and round on very curly hair.

Short uniform layers are a classic modern look for both men and women.

Combinations

And there you have it — the four basic haircuts. An infinite variety of hairstyles can be created by using these four in combination with each other. In the grocery store checkout aisle, in the dentist's waiting room, or browsing at the salon, as you flip through the pages of magazines you should be able to recognize the haircuts that you see, and determine whether or not they'd work for you. You can then use this information to communicate with your hairstylist.

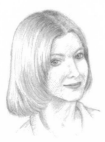

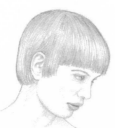

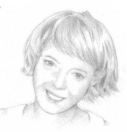

Subtle layers around the face blend into a horizontal blunt cut through the sides and back.

Highly texturized layers can fall into separate horizontal blunt-cut lines at the fringe, sides, and back.

This graduated cut combines well with layers over it. In fact, this is probably one of the most popular styles out there.

CUTTING CURLY
VERSUS STRAIGHT HAIR

I have very curly hair, so many of my clients are also curly haired. They must think I hold the secret formula when it comes to cutting curly hair! In a sense it's true, though — I've learned from my own experiences with haircuts what works and what doesn't.

Many curly heads of hair look bone straight when wet. If you have curly hair, you know that it can be significantly longer when wet than when dry. You have two options:

1. Have it cut damp. Trust that your hairstylist knows how to allow for the length reduction by taking off no more than absolutely necessary. When I cut curly hair, I begin with hair that is towel-dried and has a leave-in conditioner in it; as I cut, and the hair dries, I don't rewet it. I simply continue cutting and then texturizing as the hair's own natural growth patterns and texture start to become more evident. I also tend to cut curly hair under minimal tension so that the natural curl can "bounce" into place and is allowed for before cutting. Using tension on very curly hair can create unevenness in the finished cut.

2. Blow-dry it straight, then cut. This popular option again requires that the stylists take into account the potential length reduction once the hair dries naturally. Still, this is an excellent way to ensure a precision shape, particularly in African-American hair.

TALKING TO THE PROFESSIONALS

Keep in mind that the style you want can only be created after the hairstylist takes into consideration your own head shape, facial features, and body structure, as well as your hair's condition, diameter, textural movement, and density.

In sharing this information on haircutting, my hope is to help you approach your hairstylist with a greater knowledge of the possibilities. I've also used the terminology that's standard in salons to help you better talk to and question your hairstylist about your haircut.

CHAPTER 8

Techniques and Natural Formulas for Your Daily Styling Regimen

Having naturally healthy hair means remaining mindful of how everything you do to your hair or scalp will affect or improve their health. The more natural your approach to cleansing and conditioning, and the more you use your haircut to complement the natural features of your hair and body, the less you will have to resort to an endless variety of products and styling techniques. And which of these styling techniques and products you choose — or choose not — to use is important. The decisions you make and the procedures you use will determine whether you can have shiny, vibrant, resilient hair that requires minimal upkeep and product usage.

The important things to know about styling your hair are directly related to the result that you're looking for. One haircut can result in several dramatically different looks depending on the styling techniques that you use. Your desired look will determine your choice of styling products, tools, and procedures. Whatever the result you're aiming for, do your best to work with your hair's natural tendencies. A minimum of forceful styling encourages your hair to look its best without compromising its health or condition.

WORKING WITH STYLING PRODUCTS

There is an overabundance of styling products available out there. My first recommendation is that you see your professional cosmetologist or hairstylist for suggestions on which products you should use to create the finished style you want. The most important thing to remember is that you, yourself, need to be able to maintain the look you ask your hairstylist to give you. If your stylist begins to put styling products in your hair and works without giving you instructions, take the intiative to ask some very direct questions:

How much of each styling product should you use? Where should you apply it — near the scalp, along the complete strand, or just along the ends? Should you layer products over each other? Your stylist should be happy to explain to you the particulars of maintaining your hairstyle.

Why Use Styling Products?

Given the environmental extremes to which we expose our hair every day, without styling products it can become fly-away, frizzy, unmanageable, static prone, and much more. For this reason I usually endorse the use of some type of styling product. The holding power of a styling product will give the hair fiber more heft, body, shape, and manageability. The degree of hold necessary is determined by what you are trying to get your hair to do, the type of hair that you have, and its condition. If your hair has been cut to follow its natural tendencies, then chances are you won't need a lot of heavy holding products.

Four-Step Styling

My favorite way to approach styling products is a four-step layering process:

1. Condition. A leave-in conditioner can serve as a foundation for other products that will be used, similar to the moisturizer that you put on your face before you put on your makeup foundation. Some leave-in conditioners contain silicone to smooth down the cuticle (on the ingredients label, look for DIMETHICONE or CYCLOMETHICONE). If not, then I work a couple of drops of a silicone shiner product through the damp hair.

2. Hold. Choose a holding product appropriate for your style — soft, medium, or firm hold — in the form of liquid spray, gel, mousse, molding cream, or volumizing lotion. I have even used some of the light-hold hair sprays (what you usually use after the style is dry) to lightly apply to damp hair and blow-dry — this creates shiny, bodied hair, but you won't really feel any of the product in it.

3. Dry. After blow-drying and/or styling the hair, a light layer of hair spray may be required, depending on your hair type and style. This will give the style a "memory" of the shape you want it to hold.

4. Shine. A final light massaging or stroking of a shiner product through the hair finishes off the style.

This is the general approach for all styling. It's all a matter of degree, and also moderation.

COMMERCIAL STYLING PRODUCTS

As with shampoos and conditioners, you will find a variety of ingredients in commercial styling products that are synthetic, natural, or a combination of the two. Many of the ingredients used in shampoos and conditioners are also used in styling products — along with a completely new set of ingredients that allow the product to impart hold to the hair.

The essence of styling products is first, to give the hair a feeling of body by depositing a film over the hair strands; and second, to give "set" memory to the style by getting the hair to hold together. The amount of hold may be described as ranging from light to firm hold. Foams, gels, and lotions coat individual hair strands as well as get hair strands to "stick" together, while hair spray creates an overall or spot-specific hold over the surface area.

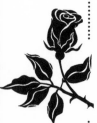

The lion's share of styling products are predominantly made of synthetic ingredients, many of which have been proven allergenic or toxic for certain individuals. Remember that these ingredients are left on, not rinsed off, and have sustained contact with the scalp. Depending on the quality of the product and the amount of polymer or resin it contains, flaking can be one of its main drawbacks. Many of the synthetic chemical ingredients can also dry the hair.

An additional concern with styling products, particularly those that contain propellants to facilitate spraying, is that these vaporous and gaseous ingredients are easily ingested into the lungs. Protect your eyes and keep your mouth closed when spraying any product onto your hair. Somewhat reassuring is the fact that advanced technology and tough environmental regulations have greatly reduced the amount of air-polluting volatile organic compounds (VOCs) in hair sprays — but you still wouldn't want to ingest them, even in small doses.

I highly recommend that you purchase *A Consumer's Dictionary of Cosmetic Ingredients* by Ruth Winter (Crown Trade Paperbacks, 1994). This book will be indispensable as you label-surf any of the personal care items that you are looking to purchase.

Styling products serve a definite purpose in giving you control of your hair and manageability; just use them in moderation. Consciously examine the products that you are going to use. Study the ingredients list. Be guided by your professional cosmetologist. Visit your whole food or health food store and examine its lines of styling products. You can cast a vote to change products for the better with your purchasing power.

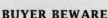

BUYER BEWARE

One of the more common ingredients seen in all forms of styling lotions, potions, and sprays is PVP/VA copolymer. This is a petroleum-derived chemical that may be considered toxic, since particles may contribute to foreign bodies in the lungs of certain sensitive individuals. In one study profiled by Ruth Winter in *A Consumer's Dictionary of Cosmetic Ingredients*, modest doses administered to rats caused the development of tumors. I recommend limiting or avoiding use of products containing PVP/VA copolymer.

FOAM OR MOUSSE

Description: Foam volumizes the hair, whether you blow-dry it smooth or diffuse it to refine and define textural movement and curls. Foam's lightweight control is great for fine hair. Conditioning foams work well for more porous, dry hair types. The label will state the amount of hold, from light to firm.

When to apply: This product spreads easily through damp hair, primarily because of how it's made: Its resins (holding ingredients) are puffed up with air. You can also spot-apply foam to dry hair for control, or to revive or change your style.

GEL

Description: Often called sculpting or molding gel, this product is traditionally used for firm hold. It is usually thick and delivers a firm-bodied hold to all hair types.

When to apply: This gel is generally used in molded or naturally dried short styles. Dry the gel into your hair while you hold it in place, or blow-dry it into short styles if you desire lots of hold and volume. Gel is usually too thick to blow-dry into longer lengths of hair.

LIQUID GELS AND STYLING LOTIONS

Description: These products come in a wide variety of types, from spray to pour on; their names range from *liquid texturizers* to *volumizing tonics.* They are in essence diluted versions of thicker gels and deliver a softer hold. But all these products do basically the same thing: provide a certain amount of bodifying and hold to the hair, while smoothing it and imparting shine. Look for a firmer holding factor if your hair is fine, or a light to moderate hold for normal to coarse hair types. Volumizing lotions are actually the best product for finer hair types — and don't forget to apply them near the scalp area in order to accentuate lift.

When to apply: Towel-dry, apply a leave-in conditioner, use a wide-toothed comb to detangle your hair, and then apply the liquid gel or styling lotion before blow-drying. You can also use these products as spot touch-ups on dry hair.

STRAIGHTENING GELS AND CREAMS

Description: These products are primarily for use on curlier or frizzier hair that is blown dry smooth. They generally have conditioning ingredients that also help control frizziness in high-humidity situations.

When to apply: Use on towel-dried, damp hair and then blow-dry to obtain the smoothest, sleekest effect possible.

MOLDING MUDS AND CREAMS

Description: These products create a buildup on the hair; indeed, that is their primary purpose. I see these as a high-fashion or special-effects type of hairstyling product. The hair takes on a laminated, coated look. Muds and creams are great for more textured cuts or hair that has textural movement. They make your hair look "lived in."

When to apply: Apply muds and creams to damp hair, ruffle through with your fingers, and then leave to dry normally or power dry with blow-dryer. You can also use them to ruffle through dry hair to "break it up."

POMADES

Description: Pomades are usually used to maintain a smooth, sleek look. These have no humectants and can add considerable weight to the hair. They will give the hair a high-gloss look and will repel moisture, preventing frizziness in high-humidity situations. They're excellent for smoothing coarse hair. Some manufacturers also produce exactly the opposite: humectant pomades for straight and curly hair that *attract* moisture to the hair.

When to apply: Smooth sparingly over dry hair.

SHINE PRODUCTS

Description: These products are non-oily and make the hair feel like silk. They work to fill any gaps in the hair strand, getting the cuticle to lay down and smoothing the hair shaft.

When to apply: Use on damp hair before blow-drying to release their lubricating qualities. Or apply them to your finished style: Spread a couple of drops between the palms of your hands, then massage them through more textured hair or smooth them over the top surface of smooth styles. Use these products in very small amounts; they can create an undesirable buildup on the hair if used excessively.

HAIR SPRAYS

Description: Primarily for holding a style in place, hair sprays can help resist humidity while deterring static. They are available in a variety of holding strengths, as well as in aerosol and nonaerosol versions. Some of the firmest sprays come in a nonaerosol form that is often referred to as spritz. Lighter-hold sprays can be used on all hair types and can easily be combed or brushed through, while spritz sprays are usually used on styles that will not be disturbed (what I have been known to call "helmet head hair"!).

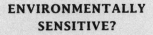

ENVIRONMENTALLY SENSITIVE?

You will notice some drastic changes in hair sprays as we head into the new millennium. Manufacturers of these products are being required by government legislation to cut back and/or eliminate their VOCs (volatile organic compounds). These propellants are proven to damage the ozone layer by releasing vapors into the lower atmosphere, thus trapping heat and ultraviolet radiation near the earth's surface.

When to apply: Hair spray is usually used as a holding product and applied to dry hair. Many of the lighter-hold sprays today can also be used as working sprays, which means that they work with the heat of the blow dryer (apply to damp hair before blow-drying). You can also spray them onto meshes of hair before you use a curling iron or hot rollers. Apply hair sprays at least 6 inches (15 cm) away from the hair to diffuse them. A concentrated blast can make the polymers and resins go on too thickly, causing a stiff, matte bond in the hair that can be unsightly.

Note: For the most healthful approach, look for hair spray products with gum arabic, gum tragancanth, and panthenol, and choose pump sprays over aerosols. Aerosols will allow very fine particles to get in the lungs, irritating them. Use caution if you spray an aerosol so you don't breathe it into your lungs or allow it to drift into your eyes.

MAKING YOUR OWN STYLING PRODUCTS

Following are some simple homespun recipes for your own styling products, or what I like to call liquid styling tools. You can create these with ingredients available from your whole food or health food store. These recipes and suggestions are simplicity itself, and all you'll need if your styling needs are minimal.

AROMA STYLE(ING)

Remember that you can distribute a wonderful fragrance through your hair by simply working a couple of drops of your favorite essential oils through your damp hair before drying. To refresh dry hair, massage essential oils through it or put a couple of drops on a brush before brushing through your hair.

ONE-INGREDIENT STYLING STANDBYS

Remember that you can use any of the old standbys discussed earlier (see chapter 6) to bodify your hair: beer, champagne, and aloe vera gel to name a few. Work any of these into shampooed, conditioned, and towel-dried hair. Adjust the amounts according to the thickness you desire. All of these ingredients contain natural sugars and proteins that will dry on the hair, leaving a film that will bodify and impart hold.

FLAXSEED GEL

This simple recipe is one of my all time favorites. It is so easy, and the resulting styling lotion is 100 percent organic and natural. The mucilaginous and emollient nature of flaxseeds makes them excellent to use as a styling lotion or gel that molds, controls, and bodifies the hair while imparting a wonderful sheen. The vodka allows the gel to dry faster as well as serving as a preservative. If your hair is drier, you can opt not to use the vodka.

2 tablespoons (30 ml) organic flaxseeds
1 cup (250 ml) purified water
1 tablespoon (15 ml) organic aloe vera gel
1 tablespoon (15 ml) high-proof vodka
3–5 drops essential oils of your choice

Yield: 5–10 applications, depending on hair length

To make:

1. Combine the flax seeds and water in a small stainless-steel or glass pan and bring to a boil, stirring frequently. Reduce the heat and simmer, uncovered, for a few minutes, stirring at intervals. Cover and let sit for 5 to 10 minutes.

2. Strain out the liquid into a glass container that can be sealed airtight. Add the aloe vera gel and vodka, then stir thoroughly. Allow to cool, then stir in a few drops of your favorite essential oils. Seal the bottle airtight. Store in a cool, dry location and use within 2 weeks.

To use:

Apply sparingly to damp hair and style. Use a small amount for light hold, more for a firmer hold. You can also use a small amount on dry hair to touch up or detail the style.

To thin or thicken: Use fewer seeds, or dilute with distilled water, to make a thinner lotion. Use more flax seeds, or substitute organic psyllium seeds, to create a thicker gel.

SUGAR-WATER HAIR SPRAY

Having lived through the punk rock era in the late 1970s and the New Wave of the early 1980s, I can vouch for this recipe. The wild hairstyles during this period were a lesson in molding hair. Mohawks and all forms of technicolor hairdos walked the streets. In London I saw firsthand the punk rock influence where it was born, bred, and evolved. All forms of flamboyant hair ruled — as did the use of sugar solutions to mold and stiffen the hair, holding it in place. A sugar-water hair spray can also be used for much more natural effects.

You may opt not to use this type of spray if your hair tends to get frizzy or affected by humidity and you'd like it to stay smooth and sleek.

1 tablespoon (15 ml)
sugar
1 cup (250 ml) hot
purified water
1 tablespoon (15 ml)
vodka (optional)
3–5 drops essential oil
of your choice
(optional)

Yield: 5-10 applications, depending on type of usage

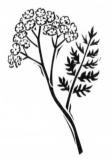

To make:
Dissolve the sugar in the hot water. Stir thoroughly to dissolve, then add the vokda and essential oil. Any leftovers should be stored in a cool, dry place and use within one week.

To use:

For setting and molding: Work this solution through damp hair for firm hold.

As a hair spray: Put the liquid in a bottle with a micromisting mechanism or in an atomizer. You will have to rinse the nozzle under hot water after each use to avoid clogs. Lightly mist your hair. When used on dry hair, this spray can be wet. Don't run your fingers or a brush through your hair until the sugar solution dries.

To thicken: Dissolve the 1 tablespoon (15 ml) of sugar in 6 tablespoons (90 ml) of hot water for a solution with more thickening power.

CITRUS HAIR SPRAY

The fragrance of this hair spray is divine. My favorite citrus for this is organic grapefruit, although you may choose to use any organic citrus fruit, or a combination. Use this hair spray for styling damp hair or for spraying on your finished dry style.

1 cup (250 ml)
    purified water
Peel of 1 medium-
    size organic citrus
    fruit (such as an
    orange, a lemon,
    or a lime) or half
    a grapefruit
½ tablespoon
    (8 ml) sugar
1 tablespoon (15 ml)
    vodka

Yield: 5-10 applications, depending on type of usage

To make:
1. Combine the water and citrus peel in a stainless-steel or glass pan. Bring to a boil, reduce heat, and simmer, stirring constantly, until the liquid starts to slightly thicken and become sticky (about 5 to 10 minutes). Strain off the liquid.
2. Add the sugar and vodka and mix thoroughly. Put into a spray or atomizer bottle. Store any leftovers in a cool dry place and use within one week.
To use:
Spray on as desired. When the solution is dry you will be able to run your fingers through your hair, but the "set" memory will remain. Use a light touch with this spray.

HERBALIZED HAIR OIL SHINE

Hair oil can control static electricity while adding hold and shine. This is particularly effective in cold-weather climates where you may go back and forth between dry forced heat indoors and the cold and dry outdoor air. In addition, a few drops of herbalized oil put onto dry, curlier, more porous hair types can provide some protection from the heat of the blow dryer (apply to damp hair). Herbalized oil can also protect hair from the sun's UV rays, and it simply makes good sense to apply it for its emollience and lubricating protection before going out in the sun.

1–2 drops of your
    favorite herbalized
    oil (see page 107)
Yield: 1 application

To use:
Rub the oil between the palms of your hands and either massage into or stroke over your finished style.

PREVENTING STATIC

Static electricity can make your hair unmanageable and can be a real nuisance. There are several ways to reduce static electricity in the indoor environment:

Humidifier. In extra-dry weather, keep a humidifier going in your home. You could also try a small indoor fountain — along with the gentle, relaxing effects of the water falling, you may experience extra humidity in the air.

Simmerpot. A pot of water simmering on the stove with potpourri or essential oils in it will add humidity and fragrance to your home.

Diffuser. An aromatherapy diffuser — you put essential oils into water, and light a tealight candle underneath — will also enhance humidity and add fragrance.

Fabric softener. To control static electricity, use a natural fabric softener in the dryer to impart emollients into your clothes. Otherwise, that fuzzy sweater, or your flannels, and even cotton will be highly charged with static electricity and in turn affect your hair. There are natural fabric softeners available at most whole food markets.

TOOLS OF THE TRADE

Let me discuss the tools most commonly used to style hair. My belief is that other than blow dryers, which I deem useful at times, all other tools should be avoided or used minimally, as they have the capacity to damage the hair if used too frequently or incorrectly. Have your hairstylist show you the most effective way to use these tools. Again, it's a matter of moderation.

Electrical Equipment

Electrically powered tools are most often used in styling techniques that require some form of heat. Because heat can damage your hair, look for tools that have a thermostatic setting and will allow you to use "low" heat when styling.

Blow dryers. These come with various attachments, nozzles, diffusers, "fingers," and so on.

Irons. These range in size from small to jumbo; in shape from round curling to serrated crimper to flat straightening varieties.

Hot or steam rollers. I prefer the velvet-covered or steam hot rollers. Use these carefully, and don't overuse or become dependent on them for your daily styling routine.

Hot sticks or benders. These are heated like hot rollers, but are long, flexible tools that you spiral longer lengths of hair around. The ends are then fastened into each other to secure.

Curling brushes. These are like curling irons with round brushes on the end. Curling brushes that heat up can be great on wavy or curly hair; they let you work through and smooth the texture without losing the fullness.

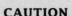

CAUTION

Great caution must be exercised when you use the kind of curling irons and straightening combs that are inserted into a hot stove. These are generally used on African-American hair, and tremendous damage can occur if they're not used correctly, as well as cumulative damage to the hair follicle over a period of time. This is due to the use of heavier oils or pomades combined with the weight of the tool and the tension used.

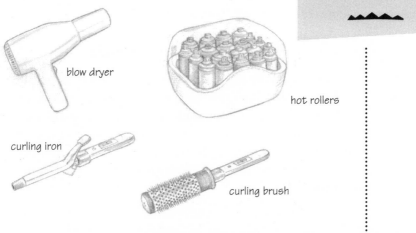

blow dryer

hot rollers

curling iron

curling brush

Nonelectric Setting Tools

Rollers: Regular, foam, self-gripping, or Velcro
Clips: Available in single or double prongs
Bobby and hair pins: To hold hair up in a style
Hair fasteners: These include combs, barrettes, fasteners, covered elastic bands

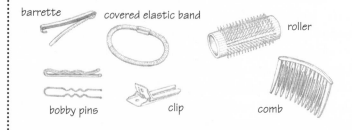

barrette · covered elastic band · roller · bobby pins · clip · comb

Combs and Brushes

Combs and brushes can help detangle and smooth your hair lengths while stimulating the scalp and promoting healthy hair growth. Use a wide-toothed comb to comb out and detangle your hair after shampooing and conditioning. Combs can also be used to smooth, direct, and detangle hair while blow-drying. They mold gelled hair into place before drying, too; comb it through again after it's dry. Use a comb with rounded teeth instead of sharp, pointed ones.

AN EASY DO

Rollers can be a great time saver in the morning ritual of styling your hair. Use them after applying a styling product and power-drying (see page 153) your hair. Put the rollers in, complete the remainder of your morning routine, and take the rollers out before you head out the door, ruffling or tousling your hair. What could be easier than that? If you have fine hair, you may want to lightly mist each mesh with hair spray before rolling it onto the roller.

Production standards. Look for combs that are "saw cut" rather than made from a mold. Saw-cut combs are made out of one piece of material; each tooth is cut out and smoothed. Combs made from a mold will have what appears to be a seam or line running down the center between the teeth. This line can cut into your hair, and the teeth are generally not smoothed.

Natural bristles or synthetic? Opinions on this issue vary. However, natural-bristle brushes have received the endorsement of the International Association of Trichologists. The natural bristle has a smoother surface and more effectively holds and distributes the hair's natural oils, leaving the hair sleek and shiny. Look for brushes with blunt-cut natural bristles that have been sheared humanely from farm-raised animals; the bristles should not be pointed or barbed. If you prefer not to use animal products, look for wood or bamboo bristles set into a natural rubber base. Such brushes are also antistatic. Some high-quality brushes combine natural and synthetic bristles. Avoid metal pins or bristles.

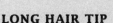

LONG HAIR TIP

The wider the spacing between the teeth, and the longer the bristles — whatever their type — the better the brush is for thick or long hair.

If you are going to blow-dry your hair, the wood and bamboo varieties are preferable — although stylists often use denman, or plastic vent, brushes, which offer good spacing between the bristles or pins and air vents for quick and efficient drying.

CHOOSING THE RIGHT BRUSH

There is no doubt about it: Brushing can damage your hair. Remember that vigorous brushing may remove some of the hair's cuticle, weakening it. So when you do use a brush, make sure it's the right tool for the job. Use it gently, and make sure it's of high quality. Poor-quality or incorrectly used brushes can do more damage than blow-drying. Of course, the right brush can also make a drastic difference in the finishing of your style. Make your selection based on your styling technique; the texture, length, and density of your hair; and the result you wish to create.

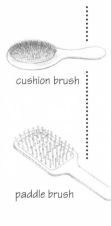

cushion brush

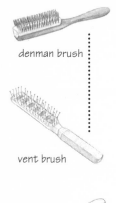

paddle brush

denman brush

vent brush

round brush

- **Cushion brushes** are oval or rectangular in shape. Preferably made of natural bristles, they are your best choice for all-over brushing of dry hair, and also excellent for the dressing or styling of long hair. The closely tufted fiber of natural bristles controls the hair and smoothes it more effectively than widely spaced bristles.
- **Paddle brushes** are usually oversize rectangular brushes. Their widely spaced bristles are well suited for drying the hair to straighten and smooth while controlling frizzies, and also for detangling long or thick hair.
- **Blow-drying brushes.** The denman brush is excellent for blow-drying sleek, smooth styles. It has several rows of plastic bristles in a rubber base. The bristles are aligned to provide excellent airflow, grip, and control. The brush head is slightly rounded, allowing you to turn it on its edges to create curves. Another blow-drying brush, the vent brush, is good for fast and gentle blow-drying because its base is thoroughly vented. This brush is at its best working through shorter styles to lift and direct the hair for volume and texture. It aerates the hair very quickly.
- **Round brushes** are also used for blow-drying, but creating smooth fullness is their primary application. These come in a variety of diameters and bristle types. The diameter you choose should be commensurate to the length of your hair and the desired results. For instance, a very small round brush would not be ideal on long hair. I recommend only the natural-bristle variety, which effectively smoothes the hair while creating volume. Very large natural-bristle round brushes are great for smoothing out frizzies and adding fullness. They're also effective for blow-drying longer lengths super straight because of the grip that they give to the hair. Metal-based round brushes conduct heat and can almost act as curling irons in some instances. Use caution with these, especially since the more delicate and "weathered" ends of your hair are closest to the heated metal core when drying.

Care, Cleaning, and Cautions

Wash your combs and brushes regularly in a gentle castile soap, but don't let them soak too long, because this could loosen the glue that holds the bristles in place. And remember, do not use anyone else's combs or brushes. A special note on this subject: Professional salons are aware of the need to thoroughly disinfect combs and brushes used on different clients. However, not all individual stylists may adhere to this. Watch carefully where the combs and brushes come from in the salon, and don't hesitate to ask your hairstylist point-blank whether they were cleaned and disinfected. Thankfully, most salons are assuredly up to snuff when it comes to maintaining high sanitation standards.

TIPS FOR USING BRUSHES

- Don't use metal bristles, which can snap and break hair strands.
- Don't use a brush to detangle wet hair — use a wide-toothed comb.
- When blow-drying, keep the brush and blow dryer in constant motion through your hair, and try to keep the blow dryer at least 6 inches (15 cm) away from it. Use a styling protectant such as a leave-in conditioner with silicone to lubricate the hair strands.
- On fine thin hair, softer bristles work best, while firmer-bristle brushes work best on thick, coarse, curly, or extremely frizzy hair.
- Choose bristles that are flexible and gentle, but still strong enough to grip the hair.
- Forget the hundred-strokes-a-day myth; this can make oily hair oilier or, in the case of dry or brittle hair, cause hair breakage.
- Keep brushes clean.
- If all else fails, remember that the best and most natural brush or comb is your fingers.

AN INTRODUCTION TO STYLING

When you're styling your hair, options range from a wash-and-wear hairdo to a blown-dry, sculpted finish. Think about the techniques you are comfortable with and the amount of time you are willing to devote to styling. Consider the volume and movement you are (or are not) attempting to create — whether and where you want your hair to be closely contoured to your head, to lift upward from the base or scalp area to create volume, or to stay flat and contoured to the head at the base area and then roll upward, creating a beveled upward effect.

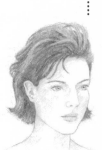

This hairstyle shows volume at the top, contoured closeness through the sides, and a beveled effect at the back.

The Natural Wash-and-Wear Styling Approach

Whether your hair is short or long, the natural styling and drying approach outlined in the steps below is the most healthful approach. Remember that damage is cumulative; prevention is the key. Indeed, we are our hair's (and skin's) own worst enemy.

Step 1: Combing out. After shampooing, conditioning, and blotting dry with a towel, use a wide-toothed comb to begin combing out your hair, working from underneath sections toward the top and from the ends toward the scalp area to detangle as needed. If you applied a leave-in protective conditioner, this combing-out process will be a breeze; the conditioner will also provide lubrication for blow-drying, protection from the sun, and insurance against color fade. Do not use a brush or pick to detangle freshly shampooed hair. These tools are too aggressive and can snap the hair.

Step 2: Towel-drying. Next, towel-dry your hair as gently and thoroughly as you can. No aggressive rubbing here! The more you can towel-dry, the less you'll need to blow-dry.

Step 3: Applying a styling product. Work your choice of liquid styling product, such as a foam, gel, or voluminizing tonic, through the hair. Remember to use it sparingly. You can always put more on, but if you apply too much your hair can look dirty and become unmanageable, greasy, or limp.

Step 4: Air-drying. There are two ways to approach air-drying, depending on your goal.

- *For texture and volume.* Gently massage the hair as it dries to help expand its shape and enhance its textural movement. You can also flip your head over and use the pads of your fingertips to gently massage at the scalp area. This allows the hair here to dry more quickly and lift out away from the scalp area.

- *For a smooth result.* Apply a styling product and then mold the hair neatly into the direction that you want it to go. Smoothly combed and distributed hair will dry smooth and sleek, while hair that has been ruffled through with a styling product will dry with more texture and retain a memory of the style that you've molded into place. You can then brush through, finger-comb, or rake through your hair to soften the look, especially if you've added gel.

Step 5: Adding more fullness and directional support. If you want to add more fullness to your hairstyle, toss your head forward and massage your scalp gently. While your head is forward, you can also apply a light hair spray over your hair from underneath; then, when you bring your head back upward, place your hair as desired, massaging the scalp with your fingertips in a rotational movement to encourage the hair to move in the desired direction. Spray over all the hair or in spot areas to add extra lift, control, and volume.

Tip: By the way, this technique — tossing your head forward and massaging your scalp — is the number one technique that I teach my clients for reviving fullness in the hair throughout the day.

If you have wavy or curly hair, don't brush or finger-rake through your hair unless you want to diffuse the texture; brushing it through can actually make it look fuzzy or frizzy. The goal with naturally dried curlier styles is to manipulate the curls as little as possible.

Step 6: Adding shine. As a final step, stroke or massage a few drops of a silicone shine product, or a drop of herbalized oil, through your hair to add a healthy radiance to the finish.

To add fullness, or to refresh a style during the day, toss your head forward and massage your scalp gently.

STYLING WITH A BLOW DRYER

Since blow-drying is the primary technique used to dry the hair today, let's look at some keys to this approach.

First, the tool itself: The crucial components for blow dryers are their temperature controls and wattage. I recommend dryers in the 1,200- to 1,500-watt range. Some blow dryers have separate temperature and air-speed controls. Generally speaking, heat forms the curl or smoothness, while cool air helps hold the styled effect in place. However, temperature controls combined with air speeds can be modulated for a variety of needs.

diffuser

finger attachment

concentrator

Blow dryers have multiple attachments for different purposes. *Diffusers* are wide dish-shaped attachments used to soften or diffuse the airflow, spreading it out over a larger area of the hair. These primarily help dry and accentuate textured, wavy, or curled styles. *Concentrators* are used to concentrate the airflow onto a small area — most often a brush that you're working through your hair to smooth the lengths. *Finger attachments* have become popular for lifting and aerating the hair. The teeth of this attachment do in essence what you can also do with your fingers.

Hair is like butter: When warmed, it can take on any shape you wish. Consider that blow-drying can take body out of your hair or put it in, depending on which techniques you use — finger-drying (massaging), diffusing, or brush-drying.

CHOOSING THE RIGHT SETTINGS

Speed	Setting	Comments
Full	Medium	Excellent for quick, efficient, no-fuss power-drying
Medium	High	Used sparingly, will smooth curls and frizziness
Low	Medium	Will "set in" waves and curls
Low	Cool	Preferred for more fragile hair types, or chemically treated hair
Low	Cool	Adds fullness to thin, fine, or sparse hair
Any	Cool	Will "set" any shape desired; some dryers also have a "cool shot" button for a quick shot of cool air

WORKING WITH A HAIR DRYER

Nothing replaces letting the hair air-dry naturally for its healthful benefits. Think about it — as soon as you apply any form of heat or forcefully pull a brush through your hair, you are breaking the hydrogen bonds that comprise the hair. Your hair already endures a lot every day — shampooing, towel-drying, exposure to the elements, and much more. Blow-drying simply adds another element of degradation to the life and health of your hair.

To alleviate some of the damage, cut down on the amount of time you spend blow-drying — you don't have to dry your hair completely — and keep the blow dryer on a cool setting. Also, use a styling protectant, such as a leave-in conditioner, which will form a protective coating over the hair strands.

Step 1: Prepare your hair. Do not blow-dry hair that is dripping wet! It's a waste of energy, yours and the power company's. Instead, thoroughly towel-dry your hair and apply a leave-in conditioner or the appropriate styling product or both to protect the cuticle layer from the heat.

Step 2: Power-drying. This technique can be the sole method used to dry the hair or simply can get rid of excess moisture before you style with your fingers or brush. Direct the airflow around your head while you massage and separate the hair with your fingers into the pattern and direction that you want it to move. If you want to smooth down your hair, this step can alleviate overbrushing and potential cuticle damage. Adjust the air-speed and temperature settings for your hair type and condition. The more textured you want your hair to ultimately look, the lower the settings you should use; otherwise you could blow your waves or curls around, making your hair look out of control or frizzy.

As you power dry, use your fingers to direct your hair in the pattern that you want it to follow.

Step 3: Styling. After power-drying has partially dried your hair, there are a variety of techniques you can use to style with a blow dryer, depending on your desired result.

- *For body and fullness,* blow-dry the base area, nearest your scalp, first, directing the air flow up and away from your head or in the direction opposite that in which you'll wear your hair. You can use your fingers or a comb or brush to lift this area. After partially drying the base area this way, blow-dry the lengths in the direction of the desired style lines. Work area by area from the sides to the top to the back.

- *For a smooth, sleek style,* direct the airflow to follow the brush direction. Work systematically with parted-out sections or panels of hair. On longer hair, use sectioning clips to hold sections up and out of the way as you dry the lengths underneath. To smooth coarse, frizzy, or curly hair, blow-dry with high heat and brush tension (the pressure you exert with the brush). Proceed with caution and limit this type of styling, because this is precisely the type of styling technique that, when used frequently, will damage your hair.

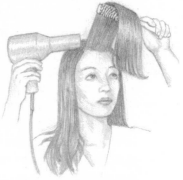

Blow-drying for a smooth, sleek style

- *To remove frizziness yet maintain body,* use minimal tension with a round brush. Remember, do not apply both heat and tension simultaneously unless you're trying to smooth and remove the texture or body from your hair.

- *To create base lift,* take a section of hair that is the width of the brush that you are using and roll the brush down to the base or scalp area so that it sits on the section, and then direct the airflow at that section. The angle of the brush will determine the volume created. The more lift you give at the base, the more volume and fullness you will achieve. To create strong base lift, consider using a comb; this is especially helpful on highly waved or textured hair where a brush is not able to work as closely or as precisely.

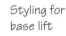

- *To create a natural, free-flowing texture,* bend your head over toward the floor after partial drying. Gently brush, comb, or simply run your fingers through your hair in this direction, directing the airflow to follow. This will give the hair — particularly limp, fine, and straight hair — more lift, bounce, and fullness while decreasing tangling, improving scalp circulation, and generally increasing volume and body. Make sure that you open up the hair and get the airflow to the base area as you're doing this. Apply a light-hold spray before you bring your head back up.

Styling for base lift

- *To create a bouncy, defined texture,* fix a diffuser attachment to your blow dryer. Apply the appropriate styling product, generally a foam, liquid gel, or volumizing lotion. Drop your head forward and cup the free-falling hair up into the dish of the diffuser, compressing the diffuser toward your head. After a few minutes, bring your head up then drop it to one side so that your hair falls freely away from it, and again diffuse. Repeat to the other side.

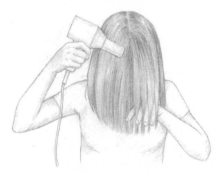

Blow-drying for a natural, free-flowing texture

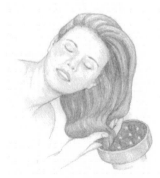

Cupping hair with a diffuser for a bouncy, defined texture

ABOVE ALL, MODERATION!

Hairstyling tools, especially those that employ heat, can give you instant volume and curl — but they can also weaken and dry your hair, as well as cause split ends. Use them in moderation and reason, and make sure that you've put a protectant on your hair before styling. Use these tools mindfully, not mindlessly, and you'll minimize the potential damage that they can inflict.

QUICK TIPS FOR HAIR HEALTH

◆ Keep in mind that any styling implements, including the blow dryer, can become tools of destruction, damaging your hair's health. To avoid this, keep the blow dryer in constant motion, and use each implement's lowest temperature settings whenever possible.

◆ Remember that a leave-in conditioner (to serve as a thermal protector) and the right choice of styling product will go a long way toward protecting your hair, particularly when you're going to do any form of heat styling.

◆ If you are "active" in your sleep, do not wear rollers or any other styling equipment to bed. This can put undue stress on the hair follicles, leading to hair breakage.

◆ Take a look at all the hair tools that you use, and get rid of any that are broken or in disrepair. This includes everything from the comb with broken teeth or brush with broken bristles that can snap hair, to the barrette that has lost its protective plastic coating.

◆ Make sure that you only use covered bands for fastening your hair into ponytails or the like. Elastic or rubber bands cut into the hair, causing great damage and excessive tension on the hair.

◆ Work with your professional stylist to develop a style that will work with, and not against, your hair's natural inclinations.

CHAPTER 9
Altered States: Color, Wave, and Relaxing Hair Treatments

▼▼▼▼▼

As you institute a naturally healthy approach to hair care, it is not absolutely necessary that you discontinue or refrain from coloring, waving (perming), or relaxing your hair to achieve a certain look. However, you should know how to minimize the risks that are involved and to control the damage. Your most important precaution is to *limit the frequency* of color or texture services, because most damage is caused by the overlapping of chemical processes within short periods of time.

However, it is important to realize the possible consequences of having chemical color or texture services done. Coloring, waving, and relaxing can be the most damaging services done to the hair — but *can be* are the operative words here. So much depends on how the process is administered and the nature of the chemical applied. As professional hair designers and their clients continue to ask for the most healthful hair care products, beauty manufacturers continue to devote tremendous amounts of time, effort, and finances to developing state-of-the-art products — and they get better all the time.

For safety's sake and to minimize the possible damage to your hair, I also recommend that you have these procedures administered by beauty professionals, who are highly qualified to perform them.

CHOOSING THE RIGHT HAIR COLOR TREATMENT

There are many types of coloring treatments available in the marketplace. Altering hair color has become a highly competitive segment of the hair care industry, with manufacturers offering everything from color mascara rinses to color glazes to semi-, demi-, and permanent treatments to henna applications. It's daunting array of choices. However, I would like to encourage the use of safer, less damaging techniques, such as temporary, semipermanent, demipermanent, and natural dyes, and discourage the use of stronger, harsher permanent, double process, and progressive dyes. The choice for you will depend on many variables, including your reasons for wanting a hair color change, the condition of your hair, and what you're willing to undertake for upkeep.

I recommend that you see your professional cosmetologist to have a color service done. There is too much that can go wrong; the amount of work done in salons to correct botched home-coloring jobs is a testament to this! Before you begin treatment, consider the following care and cautionary tips:

- ◆ Choose the most benign treatment appropriate for your situation — including a natural hair dye, if possible (see page 162). Remember, the less you process your hair, the healthier it's going to be.
- ◆ Don't stray too far from your natural level and tone. The farther you do stray, the more upkeep (repeat of application, in more frequent time intervals) will be required. If you color your hair dark blonde and naturally you are very dark brown, your outgrowth may be very obvious after 4 weeks.
- ◆ Follow your stylist's instructions for follow-up care after the treatment, and ask for recommendations for a home hair care regimen. There are many color-enhancing shampoos available to keep your color looking fresh at all times.
- ◆ Replenish your hair with protein and moisturizing treatments after any chemical coloring service.

Temporary Color

Temporary color treatments work simply by coating the outside of the hair shaft, and they last from shampoo to shampoo. Because they don't contain corrosive chemicals like ammonia or peroxide, these color treatments have no

damaging effects on the hair. They are used primarily to enhance your existing color tone — they will not change your color or cover gray. Rinses or shampoos for temporary color could be used to neutralize unwanted yellowish tones in gray hair, add highlights, or brighten your natural hair color (see Hair Color Rinses recipe on page 118).

Other products that have what could be termed a temporary effect include the wide range of color-enhancing shampoos and conditioners now available. You can also find styling products — specifically gels and mousses — that impart or accentuate tone in the hair. And coloring mascaras for the hair can be a lot of fun, creating temporary colored, highlighted effects.

Semipermanent Color

Semipermanent color treatments last through six to eight shampoos. They work by "staining" the hair shaft — the color becomes embedded in the layers of the cuticle. The more porous your hair is, or the more heat (if any) you use with the treatment, the more pronounced and durable the stain effect, especially when you are using a vibrant color tone.

Like temporary colors, damage from semipermanent colors is virtually nonexistent, although the dyes in some semipermanent treatments may have a drying effect on the outside cuticle layer of the hair. Some semipermanent color products contain dyes that can cause chemical sensitivities. Be guided by your hair colorist, or read the label if you're attempting this process on your own. If in doubt, perform a patch test (see page 93).

Demipermanent Color

Also called intermediate or deposit-only hair color, this service has become immensely popular in the salon, and it's superb for enriching your own hair color. Unlike the coating and staining effects of temporary and semipermanent color treatments, demipermanents contain an alkaline ingredient that, when combined with the developer, swells the hair shaft and opens the cuticle, allowing the color to slightly penetrate the cortex layer. Once inside the hair shaft, peroxide lifts some of the natural melanin (color) from the hair and oxidizes the artificial color molecules, making them too large to pass back out of the hair. Because it deposits inside the hair and changes the natural color, demipermanent color will have the longevity of a permanent color (4 to 6 weeks) while having less structural impact on the hair, and will gradually fade and blend with the natural color.

Colors of a More Permanent Nature

There are some chemical color treatments that can compromise your hair's health. These treatments can cause serious damage to your hair, to such a degree that it may be difficult for you to maintain the sleek, smooth, shining illusion of healthy hair. It's a matter of moderation and expertise that hinges on many factors, including the product used, the skill of your hairstylist in applying the dye, timing, the condition of your hair, follow-up care, how often retouching is done, and so on.

Permanent hair colors allow you to change your hair color in dramatic fashion, including 100 percent gray hair coverage. They work in the same manner as demipermanent color treatments, but can be more damaging.

Double-process color treatments, which involve bleaching the hair, have the potential to be the most damaging procedure possible. This type of hair color is anything but natural, and certainly not healthy for the hair.

Progressive dyes are largely marketed to men. Progressive dyes contain lead acetate (a metallic dye), which is considered a carcinogen. Lead is a systemic toxin that can penetrate the scalp and has also been proven to have adverse cumulative effects — it's even listed in the U.S. Department of Health and Human Services publication *Registry of Toxic Effects of Chemical Substances* as toxic, tumorigenic, and mutagenic! This type of color can make the hair dry and brittle. A better choice for someone who wants to progressively introduce a color change would be to have a less damaging color formula brushed onto the hair in a given percentage. This can be increased on the next visit to the salon, and so on, until the desired color has been obtained.

THE STRAND TEST

Whether you're at a salon or at home, perform a strand test before undertaking any of the longer-lasting color services, such as semipermanent or demipermanent treatments, to make sure that the resulting color is going to be what you expect and want. In the salon, we generally use a small section from somewhere in the back area of the head, where it will fall underneath; we apply the color to the strand, let it process, rinse it off, and then check the color. At home you can collect a week's worth of hairs from your brush or from shampooing. Comb through these strands and fasten one end with tape. Apply the color, process, rinse, and examine the dried color to see if it's what you were hoping for.

NATURAL, ORGANIC HAIR COLORS

Currently, there's been a major resurgence of pure vegetable hair coloring products. Primary among these is henna. Whether applied in the salon or at home, many top-quality pure vegetable hair colors and hennas are now available to color the hair. Refer to Helpful Sources for details on obtaining natural, pure vegetable dyes.

As with chemical color treatments, is very important that anyone using vegetable-based dyes also use gentle shampoos and conditioners. Protein and moisturizing treatments should be applied regularly to maintain the tone and reflective shine that the color has given and to prevent the color from fading too quickly.

Henna: The Nontoxic Approach to Hair Color

Since ancient times, the leaves and stems of the henna plant (*Lawsonia inermis*) have been used as hair cosmetics. Lawsone, the active dye principle, is found in the leaves and is used to produce a red color in the hair. A wide range of colors can be achieved, from blondes to reds to browns to blacks, by mixing the henna leaves and stems with other plant dye materials. Neutral henna, which has no coloring properties, comes from the crushed stems of the shrub and is an excellent conditioning and bodifying ingredient in shampoos and rinses. Depending on where each batch of henna comes from and when it was harvested, the strength of its properties may be subtly different.

When henna is applied to hair, it envelops and stains each hair strand, not only tinting the hair but also giving it an incredible feeling of fullness and a highly reflective shine. The results will depend on the type of henna you choose, the color, condition, and porosity of your hair, and the amount of time that you leave it in your hair. Henna is often termed a progressive dye because each additional application increases the absorption. In other words, the more often you use henna, the more penetrating the results.

USING HENNA TO COLOR GRAYING HAIR

Darker shades of henna can be used successfully on 15- to 20-percent (salt-and-pepper) gray hair to provide a blended effect. The gray hair will simply pick up tone from the henna and blend with the natural hair, to appear as if highlighted. For higher levels of gray, opt for neutral or silver henna formulas as well as the blond tones.

To cover gray, apply at the area of new outgrowth nearest the scalp for the largest percentage of time (45 minutes to 1 hour, depending on manufacturer's instructions) and work some of the henna through the ends of your hair for 5 to 10 minutes toward the end of the processing time. This works like a charm!

Henna treatments used to add tone, highlight, or enriched hair color should not be applied any more frequently than every 6 to 8 weeks, if possible. Please remember that a patch test should be done. Although henna is totally harmless, some sensitive individuals may have a skin reaction to the plant material. In addition, if you are in doubt about the color selection, I highly recommend a strand test (see page 161).

Step-by-Step Henna Application

As with all other coloring procedures, I recommend that you consult with and have your professional hair designer perform a henna treatment on your hair. Henna and vegetable hair colors are a sound and natural alternative for beautiful hair color — yet they can be unpredictable, and the coloring process can be long and messy. Your beauty professional will be able to provide this service for you with the least amount of uncertainty.

If you choose to do this color treatment on yourself, make sure that you follow the manufacturer's directions very closely.

Step 1: Liquefy the henna. Mix the henna with boiling water until it is of a smooth and creamy consistency. Three ounces (90 g) of henna, which is generally enough for shoulder-length hair, will require at least 8 to 10 ounces (235 to 295 ml) of liquid to mix thoroughly. If emollience is desired, you can add 1 tablespoon (15 ml) of olive oil to the mixture.

- To darken the tone, mix the henna with hot coffee or tea instead of water.
- To intensify the red tone, mix the henna with burgundy wine instead of water.
- To create a different color tone, create an infusion or decoction of herbs (see Henna Combinations) and use it to mix with the henna instead of water.

Step 2: Apply the paste. If you're doing this on your own, the key is to get thorough coverage. Work as neatly as possible within sections. Wear gloves so that your hands won't get stained and drape a towel around your neck to catch any drips of henna that fall. Using a broad, flat brush, work through the hair in small sections, stroking the henna paste onto the hair at the scalp and then down the strands (or just the base if you're doing a retouch).

step 2

Step 3: Secure. After applying, place a plastic bag over your hair and fasten it with a clip. You will also want to place tissue or a strip of cotton around the perimeter hairline area, so that the henna won't drip. Time according to the manufacturer's recommendations and your desired result; most treatments call for 45 minutes to 1 hour.

Step 4: Test a strand (optional). When the waiting time is almost up, you may want to check a strand of hair. Loosen one from under the plastic cap, rinse or spray it with a water bottle, and wipe off the henna with a paper towel to look at the tone. If it doesn't look ready, continue the timing process.

Step 5: Rinse, shampoo, and dry. Once the tone is to your liking, rinse thoroughly and shampoo with a gentle shampoo and a rinse-through conditioner.

HENNA COMBINATIONS

When mixed with other plant dye materials, henna treatments can produce a wide range of colors. To combine these plant materials with your henna, make a decoction or infusion, as noted (and as instructed on page 90), and substitute the herbalized liquid for the water called for in your henna formula preparation instructions. Adjust these proportions according to your desired results and the amount you need.

Plant	Part Used	Preparation Per ½ Cup (120 ml) Water	Coloring Effect
Chamomile, Roman or German	Flowers	Infusion: 2 tablespoons (30 ml)	Will accentuate honey highlights
Rhubarb	Root	Decoction: 2 tablespoons (30 ml)	Will create golden yellow tones
Saffron	Stigma from flower	Infusion: 2 grams	This may be a costly proposition, because saffron is very expensive, but it also serves as an excellent dye and will accentuate yellow
Madder	Root	Decoction: 2 tablespoons (30 ml)	Will accentuate red tones
Alkanet	Root	Decoction: 1 tablespoon (15 ml)	Will accentuate red-brown tones
Sandalwood	Heartwood	Decoction: 2 tablespoons (30 ml)	Will accentuate reddish brown tones
Rosemary	Leaves	Infusion: 2 tablespoons (30 ml)	Will accentuate brown shades
Sage	Leaves	Infusion: 2 tablespoons (30 ml)	Will accentuate brown shades
Walnut	Leaves	Infusion: 1 tablespoon (15 ml)	Will accentuate brown shades
Walnut	Husks	Decoction: 1 tablespoon (15 ml)	Will accentuate and enrich dark brown shades
Indigo	Leaves	Infusion: 1 tablespoon (15 ml)	Will accentuate lustrous blue-black tonality

WAVING AND RELAXING SERVICES

Permanent waving and relaxing services are considered texture services in today's salons. If you're facing the *daily* use of a blow dryer and a curling iron or hot rollers to achieve your desired style finish, I would consider a permanent wave or relaxing service to be a trade-off to some degree. It allows less mechanical stress on a daily basis, because your style already moves in the direction you want and has a certain amount of fullness; you don't have to achieve these every day with thermal tools, which can be harsh.

Waving or relaxing solutions open or break apart the strongest bonds in the hair, the disulfide bonds. Once broken open, these bonds shift and realign to the shape of the tool used (waving) or to a straighter, looser shape (relaxing). Great advances have been made in producing chemical formulas less damaging to hair.

Many new waving and relaxing systems have arrived in the marketplace lately, all promising a more natural and nondamaging approach. Yet one irrefutable fact remains: The means by which waves (or relaxing effects) are produced is the breaking down and reforming of bonds within the hair structure — in other words, compromising the hair's health! However, as this book goes to press, there are some revolutionary advances being made in wave and relaxing solutions that are gentle and low impact. Ask your hairstylist to keep you updated.

I strongly endorse a visit to the salon for both permanent waves and relaxers. These services involve chemicals that are toxic and should be handled only by those who are highly proficient in their usage. In addition, given the complexity of these procedures, home treatments can very easily result in overprocessed, fried hair. Professionally executed services can minimize damage to your hair, and your stylist can also guide you in the scrupulous care of your new hair texture, including which shampoos, conditioners, and styling products will complement your chemically treated hair.

Cares and Cautions
for Permanent Waves and Relaxers

If you are going to have a waving or relaxing service performed on your hair, take heed of these care and caution tips:

- I do not recommend receiving a waving process any more often than every three months; depending on your individual situation, even this might be too often.

- Don't make a drastic texture change in your hair — the greater the difference between your natural texture and the texture that is chemically waved into your hair, the more obvious the outgrowth will be. If you keep the texture change soft and natural, then your hair will be easy to handle as it grows out and you will not have to repeat the service as often.

- Make sure your hair is in optimal condition before receiving a waving or relaxing service. This will help it withstand the chemical process and come out on the other side with minimal damage. If your hair is damaged at all, it is very important that its porosity be equalized by a series of conditioning treatments and that it be fortified with protein, moisturizers, and vitamins.

- Refrain from any form of deep conditioning treatment for at least 24 hours before the waving process; it may hinder the waving process from fully taking.

- Do not brush or massage your scalp to any great degree before getting either a waving or relaxing service, as it can cause great scalp discomfort during the procedure.

- Do not shampoo your hair for at least 48 hours after receiving this service. Any aggressive treatment of the hair directly after a texture service may cause (more) damage needlessly. The bonds in the hair will not totally reform; thus the strength and elasticity of your hair will be compromised and create a dull appearance.

- Afterward, use the proper shampoos, conditioners, and styling products as recommended by your stylist to make the hair feel normal and healthy. It's not possible to fully repair the damage done to your hair — this will be removed only when the permanently waved or relaxed hair is cut away. But you will be able to fortify the hair, and make it look and feel good.
- In the retouching process for relaxing — applying relaxer to new growth — even greater damage can take place. If great care is not taken to not overlap the sodium hydroxide relaxer onto the hair that was relaxed previously, each time this overlapping takes place the hair is further weakened structurally.
- If not performed properly, relaxing has the potential to cause tremendous harm to the scalp. Burns and blisters are not unheard of. A cream protectant with a petroleum base can be applied to the scalp before the relaxer is applied to prevent problems.

PROTECTION

With all color and texture processes it is important to treat your hair as gently as possible with both the products and the styling techniques that you choose to use. And please protect your color-treated hair from the sun! Sunlight will fade your hair color quicker than you can even imagine. The sun's ultraviolet rays are detrimental even to hair that hasn't been chemically treated. The sun will have a bleaching effect on color-treated hair, as will salt water and chlorine. The best protection is to cover your hair up with a hat or scarf. You can also slick a conditioner or styling products or both through your hair to serve as protectants that contain UV filters. If you swim in a chlorinated pool or in salt water, rinse, shampoo, and condition with products for color-treated hair after your swim.

CHAPTER 10
The Salon and Spa Experience

I have spoken consistently about relying upon your professional cosmetologist, beauty professional, or hairstylist to guide you in the most healthful approach to taking care of your hair. This is more than mere lip service to my peers. Cosmetologists go through a tremendous amount of continuing education to be able to technically and creatively serve as your hair care expert. Trained cosmetologists can not only advise their clients about the best style options, but also diagnose hair and scalp conditions and prescribe a hair care regimen that is going to maintain the most healthful state for your type of hair and scalp.

FINDING AN EXTRAORDINARY SALON AND COSMETOLOGIST

As in all of life, relationships are what the beauty profession are all about. It is a service industry — we as beauty professionals are here to take care of you, and make you feel good not only about your hair but also about yourself. In a subtle way, we are healers.

Your relationship with your hairstylist can be an important piece of how you feel about yourself. To optimize the way you look and the way you feel about yourself, you want to find an extraordinary salon, one which, from the first phone call to the finishing touches, encourages a strong, healthy relationship between your body, mind, and spirit.

1. First contact. Much of your initial reaction to a cosmetologist is a result of your engagement by the salon — its sounds, sights, smells, decor; in essence, its energy. This happens from the first contact, whether it be the telephone call you make to set up an appointment or your first step into a walk-in salon. Is the experience pleasant? Does the salon receptionist or coordinator do everything possible to accommodate your schedule? When you ask about the services and prices, do you get a clear and polite response?

2. The waiting period. Once you're at the salon, is the waiting period minimal? If not, why? A wait of any longer than 10 to 15 minutes may be deemed unacceptable. Please understand that many times a stylist's schedule may be completely thrown off by an unforeseen incident or a previous client arriving late; still, this is not a satisfactory reason to cause you to be delayed. If you cannot afford a wait, call your salon shortly before your appointment to check on your stylist's time. And in turn please afford your stylist the consideration of calling to cancel well ahead of time, or if you're running late, to verify that they will still be able to accommodate you.

3. The atmosphere. Sometimes you simply may not care if you have to wait, particularly if the salon's waiting area offers your favorite magazine, videos, and organic tea or fruit juice. Some salons also offer services during a waiting period, such as a hand or scalp massage. This is the ultimate in client care!

Observe the salon while you wait. If music is playing, is it modulated to a comfortable level? Do the work and waiting areas look and smell clean? Is the air free of any intense chemical smells? As you may know, there are some highly noxious salons out there. I was once in a salon permeated by the smell of acrylic nails. I only stayed for an hour, but I came out with my head throbbing. I can't imagine how those working inside could bear it for a full workday. Progressive salons today know the importance of optimized ventilation systems.

4. Your first consultation. The consultation with a new stylist begins from the moment you meet each other with his or her handshake, smile, and simple ability to make you feel good. Ask yourself: Is the initial meeting with your hairstylist comfortable? Do you feel this person is unrushed and tuned in to you and what you are saying?

Everything that is going to take place during the service should be explained to you. As a beauty consultant, I ask very leading questions to initiate a conversation with my clients. The most important questions I ask are "What do you like about your hair?" and "What do you dislike about your hair?" And of course I always, always ask what they are willing or able to do in styling their hair on their own at home. The answers to these questions, as well as a consideration of all the hair attributes I've discussed earlier, will tell me how to approach the cutting and styling of their hair.

I touch their hair, feeling and moving it around to study its natural growth patterns, knowing that the hair's natural motion will determine a great deal about the haircut. I recommend that for your first meeting with a stylist, you go into the salon with your hair air-dried — not freshly shampooed and still wet — with as little product on it as possible, if any at all, because it is very helpful for your stylist to see your hair in this state. I prefer to see my clients as they walk in off the street, as their street clothes can speak volumes about their personal sense of style. For example, I would approach the style decision for someone who walked in with a lace blouse, pearls, and heels very differently than for someone wearing a tie-dyed T-shirt, jeans, and gym shoes, or someone wearing khakis, a sweater, and loafers. I think you get the idea.

PICTURE PERFECT?

A word here on bringing a photo to the salon to show your hairstylist. Do you want your hair to look like that model's hair, or do you want to look like that model? Aha! This is the question to be answered.

Some stylists appreciate the gesture, others despise it. If you present the photo to the stylist as an idea that you are thinking of, and do not demand that the hairstyle in the photo be replicated exactly, it should not be a problem. It is important to understand that the hairstyles on celebrities or models in many of the magazine photos that you see have been created by professional stylists and makeup artists and photographed by professional photographers. A qualified stylist will be able to look at a photo and ascertain whether the featured hairstyle can be adapted for you, and personalize it for your needs. Certainly your best approach would be, "I brought in this picture to show you a style that I really like. Do you think this will work on my hair?"

5. Discussing your options. The initial consultation — meeting your stylist, discussing your hair's natural tendencies, and determining what best exemplifies your sense of style — will help you determine the right cut and style for you. Be very specific about what you want your hair to do. If you don't know what you want your hair to do, or don't know what it can do, then express this to the hairstylist, who should be able to come up with some ideas.

Your stylist should be able to explain in an easily understandable way what he or she envisions for you, or would like to create. Before beginning, I ask my clients to *paraphrase back to me* what they understood my suggestions to be for their hair. If they say anything that indicates that they did not understand any part of the process, I take the time to clarify, so that we are both in complete understanding of what is to be done. If your stylist does not ask for this, offer it up.

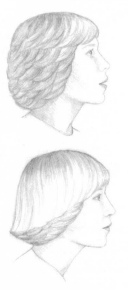

"Feather back" could be interpreted as layering through the sides (top) or stacked-out gradua-tion (bottom). Be sure you and your stylist are clear about your wishes.

Terminology in the cosmetology profession can get a little tricky at times. For example, if you tell the stylist that you want your hair to "feather back" on the sides, it is important to clarify whether "feather back" means layering throughout the sides, where more length and weight are removed, or cutting in a short graduated shape that flows back in a streamlined fashion, with stacked-out graduation that, when blow-dried, may indeed "feather back." A style selector book in the salon may help clarify — you can point to shapes, lengths, colors, and textures that you like.

Many of you see a stylist who takes care of all your hair care needs. However, if you visit a salon where chemical service specialists are responsible for any color or texture services, and the haircutter or an assistant is responsible for the cutting and styling of your hair, it is important that all these professionals confer on their vision for your finished style; everyone should be on the same page. You should all come together at some point to confirm the direction to be taken, and at that time you can hear and confirm the way your stylist communicates this direction.

6. The shampoo. For many, this is one of the best parts of the salon visit. A relaxing shampoo experience will include an all-over massage of the scalp — and a rinse that is thorough without getting your back wet! The salon should have ergonomically correct shampoo chairs, which are quite comfortable for your back and neck.

If the shampoo is rushed or uncomfortable, or if soap residue is left in your hair, either speak up and express your displeasure or determine whether you are willing to endure this on return visits. You might discreetly share this information with the salon coordinator or the stylist so that the situation can be remedied. Your input will be greatly appreciated and you will be doing a service to the salon. (This goes for any unpleasantness that you may experience. The salon management wants to hear from you!)

7. The haircut. As you're having your hair done, you'll be able to observe and assess your stylist's level of expertise. A good and highly professional hairstylist will work systematically and neatly to make the entire process a pleasure for you. He or she will work gently with your hair or move your head into required positions, being very sensitive to your comfort. You can also expect the stylist to discuss your hair and its needs with you during this time.

If the stylist is heavy handed, leaves wet hair hanging in front of your face, works in a messy or disorganized way, or in essence is insensitive to your comfort, proceed with caution. I have a very tender scalp and am exceptionally tuned in to every movement that takes place on my head. Speak up if you are uncomfortable in any way.

HOW DO YOU FIND A GOOD SALON?

I've been asked this question many times. My recommendation is to make an appointment for a manicure or a scalp treatment — any quick, half-hour treatment. While there, examine every facet of the salon. Observe the stylists working, check out the service menu, and ask the receptionist about the stylists and their specific expertise. If you get great vibes from your short visit and have all your questions answered satisfactorily, book an appointment right then and there for your return visit. A good time to go to observe is on a Friday or Saturday, when most if not all of the salon's stylists will be working.

IT'S ABOUT INFORMATION

Throughout the entire service, you should expect the stylist to share information with you, in essence educating you about what is being done and why — particularly when it comes to styling. If the stylist is not sharing this information with you, then you are not receiving the full service. It might be something as simple as the specific placement of a styling product or the way in which fingers or brushes are used to finish your style, but it could be the missing link to re-creating the magic of the salon treatment.

8. Finishing touches. After the haircut and styling treatment, you should find yourself thrilled with your style and the service you received. Your stylist should then escort you to the front reception desk to make sure that you know which products were used to create your hairstyle, and to have the receptionist bring your visit to a close, which includes booking an appointment for your next visit. I strongly endorse this planning-ahead approach, because then you know that your hair is always going to look its best. If you wait until your hair is in desperate need, chances are that you may not be able to get in to see your favorite stylist.

With a handshake or hug and a smile, you'll bid your stylist good-bye and walk out into your world with great-looking, healthy hair — hair that is silky and shiny, full of movement and energy!

THE EVOLVING SALON INDUSTRY

Salons are changing with the times. Today's beauty salon is a far cry from the salon that I worked in when I was fresh out of beauty school. I worked for a mom-and-pop business, where the money from the services was kept in my drawer with receipts until the end of the day. Today, salon management has evolved to a very high level of professionalism and offers an ever-increasing array of services.

Toxin-Free Salons

I have had the great pleasure of meeting and speaking at length with Denise Santamarina, the owner of Natural Nouveaux, a salon in Las Vegas. Denise's salon is truly toxin-free. It has to be — she was diagnosed with multiple chemical sensitivities that sidelined her from the beauty profession for a while (during which she went through an extensive detoxification program). It is an absolute necessity that everything that she uses in her salon be pure and natural. From the henna color, to the vegetable enzyme texturizing services, to the mayonnaise conditioning treatments, this salon is the real deal. In turn the salon has gained a well-deserved reputation for its uncompromising integrity. Clients who have experienced similar sensitvities are gravitating here (locally and from afar) to the point that Denise is starting to create a national reputation. Editors from magazines such as *Self* and *American Health* are calling for interviews.

Many of us are now seeking a more natural and pure way of living — one that does not use chemicals to get the job done. Denise is an inspiration, and I would love to see her bring her message to the masses, particularly in the beauty profession — to let us know that it is indeed possible to serve the needs of the clientele in a salon while maintaining the most holistic and healthful approach. Mark my words — you will soon start to see this type of salon springing up around the country. Very exciting and timely indeed!

Day Spas

Many salons are reinventing themselves as day spas by offering a full menu of body- and skin-care treatments as well as de-stressing services. Many of these salon/spas blur the lines among the medical, fitness, and beauty communities, introducing a comprehensive, holistic approach to beauty and wellness. In some metropolitan areas huge salon/spas are opening that actually have licensed medical professionals and practitioners of alternative healing arts operating their offices on the premises. From mammograms to massage to yoga to haircuts — synergy in action! Imagine, if your beauty

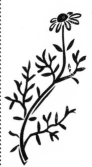

professional noticed a mole on your neck, he or she could recommend you see the resident dermatologist to have it checked out, who might recommend having it removed and send you to the resident herbalist for some postsurgery, skin-soothing herbal salves. Some very savvy salons have also set up and liaisoned

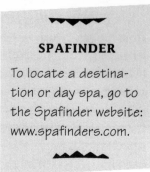

SPAFINDER

To locate a destination or day spa, go to the Spafinder website: www.spafinders.com.

with healthcare professionals in their community to provide wonderful networking and referral capabilities.

This is all happening right now in salons and spas around the country. This growing trend points out the incredibly complementary natures of beauty and wellness, and the advantages of a holistic approach to body care. In these holistic environments, all of your beauty and wellness needs can be administered to — Energy Centers, if you will. If there's not one in your local community, you may have to travel a bit farther up the road, but it is well worth it!

Now, a spa cannot replace a licensed healthcare professional's expertise. However, a visit to a salon/spa where you receive a wide variety of pampering, soothing, de-stressing services that help you feel good about yourself will serve as a preventive, synergistic measure toward good health.

A Synergistic Approach to Beauty and Health

The evolution of the salon industry is more than a fad — it is a continuing and exciting process! Full-spectrum fitness — of body, mind, and spirit — is where we are heading as we enter the new millennium. We are spiritual beings here having human experiences. Indeed, a visit to a holistic salon, day spa, or even destination (week-long retreat and rejuvenation) spa where you are able to energize, de-stress, and simply get in touch with your inner self while having someone administer to the beautifying rituals that will make you feel and look fresh and vital — this is my idea of loving and pampering yourself.

A friend of mine, a very special lady who is in remission from breast cancer, has committed herself to visiting a destination spa outside of Chicago called the Heartland Spa. She stays there for a week at a time and simply takes time to pamper her body, her mind, and in essence her soul. She disconnects from her hectic work schedule and makes time for herself. We all can learn a lesson from this. Renewal and rejuvenation can increase self-knowledge; we can then move back into our field of activity with every fiber of our being enlivened. We have taken the time to connect with our higher consciousness in a meaningful way — one that affects our health on all levels.

SPIRIT AND BEAUTY

When you know, honor, and respect yourself, you live your life in an enlightened state of being, a state that encourages you to evolve toward joy, vitality, energy, creativity, peace, and wisdom. Realizing that this is the core desire of your being for all that you experience, health and balance of your body, mind, and soul can become your reality.

The outward expression of this evolution toward enlightenment is health — healthy hair, skin, and nails, as well as a spring in your step, a smile on your face, a sparkle in your eyes, and a melodic lilt in your voice. Remember that you are a choice maker — you are making the choices that are the most evolutionary for you. Live in the present moment, and cultivate a sense of awareness, to experience not only naturally healthy hair but also a life filled with wonderment, open to the infinite possibilities that life has to offer us.

> *Go confidently in the direction of your dreams.*
> *Live the life you've imagined. As you*
> *simplify your life, the laws of the universe*
> *will be simpler.*
>
> — Henry David Thoreau

SUGGESTED READING

Ackerman, Diane. *A Natural History of the Senses.* New York: Vintage, 1990.

Chopra, Deepak. *Ageless Body, Timeless Mind.* New York: Harmony Books, 1993.

Facetti, Aldi. *Natural Beauty.* New York: Fireside, 1991.

Frawley, David, and Vasant Lad. *The Yoga of Herbs.* Santa Fe, N.M.: Lotus Press, 1986.

The Hair and Scalp. Sydney, Australia: International Association of Trichologists 1993.

Hampton, Aubrey. *What's in Your Cosmetics?* Tucson, Ariz.: Odonian Press, 1995.

———. *Natural Organic Hair and Skin Care.* Tampa, Fla.: Organica Press, 1987.

Hoffman, David. *The New Holistic Herbal.* Rockport, Mass.: Element, 1990.

Lad, Vasant. *Ayurveda: The Science of Self Healing.* Wilmont, Wisc.: Lotus Press, 1984.

Lust, John. *The Herb Book.* New York: Bantam, 1980.

Mindell, Earl. *Earl Mindell's Herb Bible.* New York: Fireside, 1992.

Monte, Tom, and the editors of *Natural Health* magazine. *The Complete Guide to Natural Healing.* New York: Perigee Books, 1997.

Murray, Michael, and Joseph Pizzorno. *Encyclopedia of Natural Medicine.* Rocklin, Calif.: Prima Publishing, 1991.

Raichur, Pratima, with Marion Cohn. *Absolute Beauty — Radiant Skin and Inner Harmony through the Ancient Secrets of Ayurveda.* New York: HarperCollins, 1997.

Rama, Swami, Rudolph Ballentine, and Alan Hymes. *Science of Breath.* Honesdale, Penn.: The Himalayan Institute of Yoga Science and Philosophy, 1981.

Sachs, Melanie. *Ayurvedic Beauty Care.* Twin Lakes, Wisc.: Lotus Press, 1994.

Salinger, David. *The International Association of Trichologists Guide to Hair Loss.* Sydney, Australia: International Association of Trichologists, 1995.

Simon, David, M.D. *The Wisdom of Healing.* New York: Harmony Books, 1997.

Sivananda Yoga Vedanta Center. *Yoga Mind & Body.* New York: Dorling Kindersley, 1996.

Smeh, Nicholaus J. *Health Risks in Today's Cosmetics.* Garrisonville, Va.: Alliance Publishing Company, 1994.

———. *Creating Your Own Cosmetics Naturally.* Garrisonville, Va.: Alliance Publishing Company, 1995.

Vogel, H. C. A. *The Nature Doctor.* New York: Instant Improvement, Inc., 1991.

Winter, Ruth. *A Consumer's Dictionary of Cosmetic Ingredients.* New York: Crown, 1994.

Worwood, Valerie Ann. *The Complete Book of Essential Oils and Aromatherapy.* San Rafael, Calif.: New World Library, 1991.

HELPFUL SOURCES

Associations and Organizations

The American Academy of Dermatology
930 Meacham Rd.
Schaumburg, IL 60173-4965
847-330-1230
Web site: www.aad.org
Offers referrals to dermatologists in your area.

The American Hair Loss Council
401 North Michigan Ave.
Chicago, IL 60611
312-321-5128
Offers educational services, referrals, and products.

The American Herbalists Guild
P.O. Box 70
Roosevelt, UT 84066
435-722-8434
Offers a directory of peer-reviewed professional herbalists; call or write for directory cost.

The Herb Research Foundation
1007 Pearl St., Suite 200
Boulder, CO 80302
303-449-2265
Web site: www.herbs.org

The International Association of Trichologists
185 Elizabeth St.,
  Suite 919
Sydney, NSW 2000
Australia
2-267-1384

In the United States, address requests for information to:
37320 22nd St.
Kalamazoo, MI 49009
Fax: 616-372-3224
For issues dealing with the scalp and hair thinning, as well as loss. Trichological procedures, therapies, and how to locate a certified trichologist.

The Look Good, Feel Better Program
800-395-LOOK
Or call your local chapter of the American Cancer Society
For women undergoing chemotherapy and radiation treatments. Professionals in the beauty industry teach cancer patients a variety of techniques to overcome the appearance-related side effects of chemotherapy and radiation treatments, including hair loss.

The National Association for Holistic Aromatherapy
836 Hanley Industrial Ct.
St. Louis, MO 63144
888-ASK-NAHA
A nonprofit educational organization.

Mail-Order Suppliers

High-quality health food stores today carry a wide selections of herbs and natural products. However, if there are no local suppliers in your area, try any of the following mail-order sources.

Ayurvedic Health and Beauty Care Products

Bazaar of India Imports, Inc.
1810 University Ave.
Berkeley, CA 94703
510-548-4110

The Chopra Center for Well Being and Infinite Possibilities International
7630 Fay Ave.
La Jolla, CA 92037
888-424-6772
Web site:
  www.chopra.com
Catalog of products, books, tapes, teas, herbs, essential oils, and more. Also offers educational courses and programs in mind-body healing and Ayurveda.

Devi, Inc.
P.O. Box 377
Lancaster, MA 01523
800-237-8221
Carries Shivani Ayurvedic Beauty Care.

Maharishi Ayur-Ved International
417 Bolton Rd.
P.O. Box 541
Lancaster, MA 01523
800-843-8332 (information)
800-255-8332 (orders)

Tej Beauty Enterprises, Inc.
162 West 56th St., Rm. 201
New York, NY 10019
212-581-8136
The location of Pratima Raichur's world-renowned Ayurvedic Beauty Salon. She is also the creator of the Bindi line of cosmetics.

Herb Suppliers

Avena Botanicals
219 Mill St.
Rockport, ME 14856
207-594-0694

Catskill Mountain Herbs
P.O. Box 1426
Olivebridge, NY 12461
914-657-2943

Frontier
Box 299
Norway, IA 52318
800-669-3275

Golden Cabinet Herbs
2019 Sawtelle Blvd. West
Los Angeles, CA 90025
800-540-6330
Chinese herbal formulas; call for a catalog.

Green Mountain Herbs, Ltd.
P.O. Box 2369
Boulder, CO 80306
800-525-2696

Herb Pharm
347 East Fork Rd.
Williams, OR 97544
800-348-HERB

Herbal Healer Academy
H.C. 32, Box 97-B
Mountain View, AR 72560
870-269-4177
Web site:
  www.drherbs.com
This company has everything you might need for your herbal pursuits, including a naturopathic doctor for consultations and hair analysis.

Healing Spirits
9198 State Route 415
Avoca, NY 14809
607-566-2701

Lotus Light
P.O. Box 2
Wilmot, WI 53192
414-862-2395

McZand Herbal, Inc.
722 14th St., Suite 230
Boulder, CO 80306
800-371-8420
Web site: www.zand.com

Mountain Rose Herbs
85472 Dilley Lane
Eugene, OR 97405
800-879-3337

Wild Weeds
1302 Camp Weott Rd.
Ferndale, CA 95536
800-553-9453
Fax: (800) 836-9453

Essential Oils Suppliers

Aroma Vera
3384 South Robertson
  Place
Los Angeles, CA 90034
800-669-9514

Auroma
1007 West Webster Ave.
Chicago, IL 60614
800-327-2025
Web site:
  www.auroma.com

Oshadi Essential Oils
Joint Adventure
800-898-PURE
E-mail:
  Aromaya@aol.com
Web site: www.access-
  newage.com/aroma

Tisserand Aromatherapy
P.O. Box 750428
Petaluma, CA 94975-0428
707-769-5120
Fax: 707-769-0868
Also at select health food stores.

Natural Hair and Beauty Products

Many of the companies listed here distribute products through health food stores, so check with your local supplier first.

Alba Botanica Cosmetics
P.O. Box 1858
Santa Monica, CA 90046
213-451-0936
A variety of personal care and cosmetic products.

Aubrey Organics
4419 N. Manhattan Ave.
Tampa, FL 33614
800-AUBREY-H
Web site: www.aubrey-organics.com
Personal care products, also available in select health food stores.

Colora Henna through Colora, Inc.
217 Washington Avenue
Carlstadt, NJ 07072
800-989-0969
Top-quality henna.

Earth Science, Inc.
620 North Berry St.
Brea, CA 92621
800-222-6720
Complete line of personal care products.

From Nature With Love
P.O. Box 201
Hawleyville, CT 06440
800-520-2060
203-270-9999
Email: information@from-naturewithlove.com
Web site: www.fromna-turewithlove.com

Herbaceuticals
902-M Enterprise Way
Napa, CA 94588
800-462-0666
Developers of NATUR-COLOR, an herbal-based permanent hair color gel; also available at select health food stores.

Jeanne Rose Herbal Bodyworks
219A Carl St.
San Francisco, CA 94117
415-564-6785
Ask for their great catalog.

Kiehl Pharmacy
109 Third Ave.
New York, NY 10003
Great hair and skin products, also bulk herbs, essential oils, and hennas; also available at select health food stores.

Liberty Natural Products
8120 SE Stark St.
Portland, OR 97215
503-256-1227
Offers a variety of herbal extracts, essential oils, and natural products.

Logona Kosmetik Pure Vegetable Hair Colors
554 Riverside Dr.
Ashville, NC 28801
828-252-1420
A full line of personal care items; also available at select health food stores.

The Somerset Company
P.O. Box 213
Bellevue, WA 98009-0213
888-449-1979
Web site: www.somer-set-co.com
Natural hair care products as well as ingredients to make your own hair care products.

Vita Wave Products, Ltd.
P.O. Box 5206
Ventura, CA 93005
805-981-1472
Vitawave offers one of the most natural permanent wave/relaxer products, as well as permanent hair color and vegetable hair colors.

Weleda
841 South Main St.
P.O. Box 769-HFB
Spring Valley, NY 10977
914-356-4134
One of the purest product lines in the marketplace; also available at select health food stores.

Yoga Resources

Living Arts
P.O. Box 2939, Dept. YJ501
Venice, CA 90291
800-254-8464
Web site: www.living-arts.com
For top-quality yoga videotapes.

INDEX

Horsetail *(Equisetum arvense)*, 91, **104,** 107, **111,** 113
Humectants, 70, 74, 79, 100, 123

Indigo, **165**
Infusions, 90, 110, 113
Insulin, 28, 60–61
Irons, curling/straightening, 145, *145*
Itchy scalp. *See* Sensitive scalp or skin

Jasmine essential oil, 95–96, **104, 111,** 120
Jojoba oil, 86, **103, 111,** 120
Juniper essential oil, 96, **104**

Kaphas, 32, 33, **34,** 43, 48, 55–58
Kidneys, detoxification of, 22–23

Labels, 67–77, 85, 105
Lavender *(Lavandula officinalis)*, 91, **104, 111,** 113, 117
Lavender essential oil, 96, **104,** 114, 115, 118, 119
Leave-in conditioners, 67, 82, 121, 135, 156
Lecithin, 69–70, 87, 100, 111, **111**
Lemon, **104,** 114, 119, 122
Lemon essential oil, 96, **104**
Lemongrass *(Cymbopogon citratus)*, 91, 96, **104, 111,** 113
Length of hair, 7–8, *8,* 125–127, *127*
Licorice, 22
Lotions, 88, 138
Lubricants, 70, 71, 79, 85

Madder, **165**
Manageability of hair, 63, 116, 143–144
   conditioners for, 121
   emollients for, 69
   rinses for, 100, 112
Marjoram essential oil, 97, **104**
Marsh mallow *(Althea officinalis)*, 91, **104,** 113
Mature skin, essential oils for, 95–99
Mayonnaise, 100, 122
Meditation, 44–46
Medium hair, 18, 78
Milk, 101
Mineral oil, 69, 85
Minerals, 52–53, 86, 87, 91, 92, 99
Mint *(Mentha* spp.), 91, **104,** 113, 118, 119
Moisture in hair, 14, 16, 79

Moisturizers, 63, 70–71. *See also* Emollients; Humectants
   conditioners, 66, 119–120, 123
   essential oils, 99
   food stuffs, 99–101
   herbs, 88
   plant oils, 85–87
   rinses, 116
   shampoos, 65
Molding products, 138, 141–142
Mousses, 137
Mucilaginous herbs, 22, 89, 91, 141
Muds, molding, 138

Natural ingredients, 63–64, 67, 72, 75–77. *See also* Essential oils; Herbs; Plant oils
   color treatments, 162–165, *164*
   foodstuffs, 99–101, 122–123 (*See also* Vinegar)
   styling products, 140–144
Neroli essential oil, 97, **104**
Nettle *(Urtica dioica)*, 91, **104, 111,** 114, 115
Neurodermatitis, 83
Nitrosamines. *See* Cancer
Normal hair and scalp, 77, 78, 80
   beneficial ingredients for, **103–104**
   essential oils for, 94, 96, 98–99
   rinses, 112, 113, 114
   shampoos, 65, **111**
Nutrition, 49–61

Oil treatments, 67, 105–108
Oily hair and scalp, **34,** 77–80, 80
   beneficial ingredients for, **103–104**
   essential oils for, 93–99
   food stuffs for, 101
   hyperthyroidism and, 28
   oil treatments, 105
   overcorrecting for, 23–24
   rinses, 99, 112, 113, 114
   shampoos, 65, **111**
Olive oil, 71, 72, 86, **103**
Orange essential oil, 73, 97, **104, 111**
Oregano *(Origanum vulgare)*, 92, **104,** 117, 121
Organic products, 23, 60, 64, 85, 93, 99–101
Ovaries, 28

Pancreas, 28
Panthenol, 70–71, 72, 121
Parabens, 71, 73
Parsley *(Petroselinum crispum)*, 92, **104**

OTHER STOREY TITLES
YOU WILL ENJOY

The Essential Oils Book: Creating Personal Blends for Mind and Body, by Colleen K. Dodt. Discusses the many uses of aromatherapy and its applications in everyday life. Includes simple recipes that anyone can make from ingredients available at health food stores or herb shops. 160 pages. Paperback. ISBN 0-88266-913-3.

The Herbal Body Book: A Natural Approach to Healthier Hair, Skin, and Nails, by Stephanie Tourles. Contains more than 100 recipes to transform common herbs, fruits, and grains into safe, economical, and natural personal care items such as facial scrubs, shampoos, lip balms, powders, and more. 128 pages. Paperback. ISBN 0-88266-880-3.

The Herbal Home Spa: Naturally Refreshing Wraps, Rubs, Lotions, Masks, Oils, and Scrubs, by Greta Breedlove. Easy-to-make recipes using herbs, fruits, flowers, and essential oils for homemade health and beauty aids that pamper every part of the body from face to feet. Also offers herbal bathing rituals and many massage techniques for treating one's friends to a relaxing spa treatment. 208 pages. Paperback. ISBN 1-58017-005-6.

Natural Foot Care: Herbal Treatments, Massage, and Exercises for Healthy Feet, by Stephanie Tourles. From easy-to-make recipes for creams, lotions, and ointments to foot massage techniques, this book offers dozens of natural ways to care for feet. Readers will find tips for choosing properly fitting shoes, giving home pedicures, and treating athlete's foot and other maladies. 192 pages. Paperback. ISBN 1-58017-054-4.

Natural Hand Care: Herbal Treatments and Simple Techniques for Healthy Hands and Nails, by Norma Pasekoff Weinberg. Focusing on alternative and preventive therapies and treatments, this book offers dozens of easy-to-make recipes for cosmetic products, plus nutrition tips for healthy hands, strength-building exercises, and treaments for arthritis and other common hand ailments. 272 pages. Paperback. ISBN 1-58017-053-6.

Naturally Healthy Skin: Tips & Techniques for a Lifetime of Radiant Skin, by Stephanie Tourles. A hands-on guide to great-looking skin for readers in their 20s, 40s, 60s, and beyond. Includes dozens of healing recipes and effective treatments for common skin problems such as acne, age spots, dermatitis, eczema, hives, psoriasis, rosacea, sunburn, and more. Also includes tips for enhancing skin health with vitamins and whole foods plus the author's own daily beauty rituals. 208 pages. Paperback. ISBN 1-58017-130-3.

The Natural Soap Book: Making Herbal and Vegetable-Based Soaps, by Susan Miller Cavitch. Provides basic vegetable-based soap recipes along with ideas on scenting, coloring, trimming, and wrapping soaps. 192 pages. Paperback. ISBN 0-88266-888-9.

These books and other books from Storey Publishing are available wherever quality books are sold or by calling 1-800-441-5700. Visit us at www.storey.com.